AN INTRODUCTORY GUIDEBOOK OF

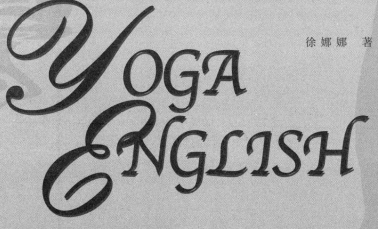

YOGA ENGLISH

徐娜娜 著

瑜伽英语入门指南

四川人民出版社

All of us
have a dormant spark of divinity in us
which has to be fanned into flames by yoga.

—B.K.S. Iyengar

我们每个人
心中都潜藏着一粒神性的火花，
　瑜伽将它催成熊熊烈焰。

　　　　——B.K.S. 艾扬格

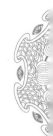

Recommendation

The author has worked diligently to compile an impressive amount of information that will help Yoga instructors and students alike. The text is clear and easy to understand broadening the Yoga instructor's ability to reach a wider group of students.

Linda Carder

USA

As a yoga teacher with 17+ years of teaching experience in China, I come across many practitioners, and Nandini is one of them. Nandini is not only a dedicated practitioner but also a seasoned translator for many renowned yoga Gurus. Her new bilingual book not only offers a comprehensive exploration of yoga, but also serves as a valuable tool for Chinese yoga practitioners to embrace yoga with a global perspective.

N.K. Singh

OM Shiva Yoga, Beijing

This book, authored by Nandini, is an invaluable resource for yoga teachers seeking to teach and learn yoga in English. I highly recommend it to teachers who wish to enhance their knowledge and proficiency in both yoga and yoga terminology in English.

Yogacharya Ashish Bist

Rishikesh, India

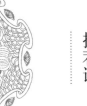

推荐语

作者努力编纂了大量将助益于瑜伽教练和学生的信息。本书内容清晰易懂，扩大了瑜伽教练吸引更广泛学生群体的能力。

琳达·卡德尔

美国

作为在中国拥有17年以上教学经验的瑜伽教师，我接触过许多中国的瑜伽练习者，其中包括Nandini。Nandini不仅是一位专注的瑜伽练习者，还是一名经验丰富的译者，担任过多位知名瑜伽大师的译员。她的双语新书不仅对瑜伽进行了全面的介绍，更为中国瑜伽练习者打开全球视野提供了宝贵工具。

N.K. 辛格

北京　印梵西瓦瑜伽

这本由Nandini编写的书对于希望用英语教授和学习瑜伽的瑜伽教师来说是一份宝贵的资源。我强烈推荐给那些希望在双语瑜伽及瑜伽术语方面增进知识和熟练度的教师。

瑜伽大师 Ashish Bist

印度　瑞诗凯诗

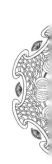

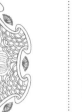

Foreword

Yoga is a gift. It is a blessing for all. It has been so for a very long time.

Small clay statues of people practicing yoga postures have been discovered in what is now Northern India. They date back around 5,000 years. One of the first known written records of traditional yoga, *The Yoga Sutras of Patanjali*, is thought to date back around 2,500 years. In this treatise, Patanjali documents the knowledge of yoga at the time. He clearly describes the meaning and purpose of yoga, and the obstacles to be overcome during practice. And he introduces the Eight Limbs of yoga: the 8 different stages of practice that can enable those who choose to practice to rise to their highest possible level of potential on all levels. Within his ancient writings are the essence of true yoga. And a path forward for growth for us all still to this day.

However, perhaps even the greatest and earliest written scriptures and teachings on Yoga have become clouded by misunderstandings that can arise through interpretation and translation difficulties. They can represent challenges that may arise when we seek to study and to learn from timeless wisdoms from different traditions written in different languages from different cultures.

In 2011, I was honoured to be invited to teach yoga and meditation throughout different yoga centres around China. Although originally intended to be for just 3 months, I continued to do this for another 7 years. Although my knowledge and experience with teaching and practicing yoga and meditation were extensive, I could not speak, read, or write Chinese. I thought I could try to learn to speak Mandarin. To be able to teach in Mandarin. But it soon became obvious that my ability to learn and understand this new language, and to be able to share yogic experiences, was far less than my ability to learn and understand yoga.

So I began to teach yoga and meditation classes around China with the help of English-speaking Chinese people. Being able to communicate now became possible with the assistance of these very patient and competent translators, and it became possible to be able to survive in China. However, I soon came to realise that being able to speak and understand English and Chinese did not mean that one could speak and understand Yoga. The yogic practices have their roots in Sanskrit language. Many of the yoga words and ideas did not have clear translations to other languages. I can remember sitting with a very competent translator discussing the subjects and meanings we would try to teach in the coming yoga class. To be told occasionally that there was no word in their language that had this meaning. It wasn' t that the translator did not know the word. There just wasn' t one. It was a yoga word.

This led me to realise that it was going to be a little more difficult for me than I had anticipated to be able to teach the subjects I had been invited to teach in a different country and in a different language. And this led to another realisation. If it was going to be difficult for me to teach these classes, it must also be quite difficult for the translator. If it was difficult for both the teacher and the translator to deliver this class, it must be extraordinarily difficult for the students to be able to understand and learn.

Without the kindness and help of translators, I could never have taught yoga and meditation in China for 7 years. I was most fortunate to be able to work with many great translators. However, it soon became obvious that teaching with a translator was not an ideal situation. I never really knew what was being said to the students. Different translators can translate different meanings to the best of their ability. It was difficult to get a feel for whether or not they, and the students, were understanding what I was trying to say. It was difficult for students to ask questions. There was this space between the teacher and the student. And this space created confusion. My Mandarin speaking abilities never became good enough to teach yoga classes in Mandarin, to my shame. Ultimately, my classes were all taught mainly in English. And to my surprise, many students who did not speak English still attended class. But I still regret not being able to share the joys and benefits of yoga with enthusiastic Chinese students in their own Chinese language.

During my time teaching in China, I came to see that the challenges I was experiencing teaching in a different language were a shared experience. As yoga becomes more popular and embraced within China, there becomes more interest and demand and need for more information and opportunities to learn. Many of the texts that are available to read from different traditions are printed in English. Many of the workshops and opportunities to study different traditions include overseas teachers who do not speak Chinese. And it was not uncommon to have overseas and Chinese students together sharing classes in many studios.

So the communication difficulties that arose through embracing new and different yoga styles and traditions was an experience shared by overseas and Chinese students, teachers, and studio owners. Not just through language differences, but also in learning new words and names for new yoga practices and techniques. Yoga words.

I remember writing out information sheets describing different aspects of meditation in English. Then I would sit with one of the Chinese students with excellent English and a kind heart and she would translate these information sheets into Chinese. That could be distributed to the students, so they may take them home to read and consider in their own time. These handouts were useful. But that is all. Then one of the translators had another idea. She could write a different yoga book for Chinese speaking teachers and students. Already there were many yoga books available in Chinese and in English. This book would be written in both Chinese and English. Each mirrored side by side on right page and left page for easy comparison. The emphasis is to be on making English language yoga information more accessible to Chinese speaking teachers and students. The book covers eight limbs of yoga, anatomy of the body, yoga terminology, step-by-step instructions for yoga poses, useful information on what happens in yoga studios, etc., with lots of informed comments and explanations that are not usually found in dry yoga commentaries. It is an idea that will help Chinese teachers and students develop and improve their yoga vocabulary and comprehension skills. All of these will lead to greater connection to the depth and wisdom of yoga experience. This book has finally been written.

If you are seeking to make the knowledge and experience of different yoga traditions more accessible, this book is for you. Wish you all enjoy and be benefited by this book.

Swami Mantramurti

Mangrove Yoga Ashram

Australia

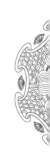

前言

随着中外国际交流增多以及国际文化传播日益加强，瑜伽逐步走入大众的视线，融入国人的日常生活中。瑜伽在中国强劲的发展势头吸引了诸多国外瑜伽大师来到中国讲学授课，国内的瑜伽爱好者也纷纷去往海外精进学习，更有不少来华工作的海外人士走入中国的瑜伽场馆进行学习。

然而，因为英语不过关，问题也随之而来：

终于得到机会和国外瑜伽大师面对面，东拼西凑的几个单词却将意思表达得支离破碎；参加价格不菲的国外名师工作坊只能依赖翻译嘴中"嚼"出来的信息，翻译质量难以保证；想潇洒地去国外学习原汁原味的瑜伽，语言这道门槛横亘在眼前；意识到瑜伽不能停留在体式上，想研读瑜伽哲学，却"啃"不动原著；馆里来了外国友人想报名学习却因语言问题产生沟通障碍……

此时，瑜伽英语的重要性你是否真切地体会到了？

在深入学习瑜伽的几年间，笔者一直在研读并收集专业瑜伽英文书籍及相关资料，并不断将积累的资源进行整理与内化，写成此书，希望您在认真学完后，能够：

1. 对瑜伽英语有较清晰与专业的认识；
2. 初步听懂国外瑜伽教师的授课内容；
3. 较为顺利地阅读通用瑜伽英语文章；
4. 运用所学初步实现双语教学或翻译。

本书首先从英语资料入手，综合多个流派的口令表达，力求英文表达地道，再结合中文教学实际做出相应调整。希望读者可以在阅读过程中勤做笔记，做好词汇表达分类，为日后设计个性化双语瑜伽课程做好准备。

Swami Satchidananda不止一次提到："Truth is one; paths are many."。意思是说，真理只有一个，而通往真理的道路却有千千万万。无论修习何种瑜伽，它都只是万千的选择之一，不是唯一。此外，我们当中有很多人沉浸在日常的瑜伽体式练习中，却很少跳出来看看瑜伽本来的样子。但我们终究要认识到体式只是瑜伽的一个组成部分，不能和瑜伽画上等号。我们对瑜伽所产生的疑惑，瑜伽经典著述早已准备好了答案，等我们去阅读，去发现。所以说，瑜伽英语不仅仅是实现双语教学的工具，它更是一把钥匙，能为我们打开一扇扇瑜伽知识之门，带我们走入更广阔的瑜伽天地。如果通过学习本书能为您探索瑜伽世界提供一点新的思路与些许助益，那我便无比欢喜了。

　　感恩瑜伽路上与您相见，愿瑜生喜乐安康！Hari Om Tat Sat.

徐娜娜（Nandini）

2020年7月

本书结构及
使用说明

瑜伽练习经由外在逐步深入到内在。因此，本书按照瑜伽自外向内练习的一般顺序进行编排。书分六章，下面作简单介绍：

第一章：瑜伽与你

第一小节主要回答三个问题：瑜伽是什么？瑜伽的目的是什么？瑜伽的流派有哪些？这些都是瑜伽学习者需要了解的最基本的问题，也是一名合格的瑜伽老师应该能够回答出的问题。

瑜伽练习的主体是个人。秉承"以人为本"的学习理念，第二小节讲解人体基本构造，包括身体部位、骨骼、肌肉、内脏器官及系统，为读者进行后续篇章的学习做好铺垫。需要说明的是，部分身体部位词汇存在不止一种表达，本书在口令部分选词尽量贴近瑜伽课堂日常用法，例如使用了shin（胫骨）而未选用tibia（胫骨）。

第二章：瑜伽体式

体式部分依据国家体育总局社会体育指导中心审定的《健身瑜伽体位标准》，从瑜伽基础体式（一至六级共108个）中选取30个，按照站立、坐立、俯卧和仰卧进行分类，将不易列入以上四类的其他常见体式列为补充类，每类使用英汉双语详细讲解6个不同难度级别的瑜伽体式。此外，附加一套完整的瑜伽拜日式口令，方便学习者在实际教学活动中灵活使用。

每个体式均附带生词表，标注了生词音标、词性、释义及词组搭配，方便读者朋友们随时查阅、积累，为学习者减轻查词负担，提高学习效率。此外，词汇索引表提供了与瑜伽教学情景相关的生词例句。读者可以通过实例掌握这些词汇在实际教学活动中的应用。在编辑本书的过程中，笔者参考对比了不同瑜伽流派的口令，力求展现多元化的语言表达方式，以提供更为丰富的语料，尽量满足读者自由选择和搭配出个性化体式口令的需求。因此，请勿使用某一流派的标准要求口令表达的规范性。为方便理解，体式中英译名采用目前国内课堂常用表达，如Utkaṭāsana中的utkaṭa在梵文中意为fierce（凶猛的，猛烈的），在本书中则取其体式形象将Utkaṭāsana译为幻椅式（Chair pose）。

第三章：瑜伽休息术

缺少休息术的瑜伽课是不完整的。这一章节首先讲解瑜伽休息术的定义、重要性以及练习的注意事项，后附完整的双语休息术引导词。瑜伽休息术框架基于Swami Satyananda Saraswati的*Yoga Nidra*（《瑜伽休息术》）一书，口令简明扼要，条理清晰，专业性较强，读者可根据个人需求进行增减用于日常教学活动中。

第四章：瑜伽调息法

本章节介绍了瑜伽调息法的定义、重要性以及练习时的注意事项，以腹式呼吸和经络清理调息法为范例，帮助读者在掌握调息法基础词汇的前提下，轻松理解并掌握调息法双语口令，顺利开展双语教学。

第五章：瑜伽冥想

冥想不仅是瑜伽会员课及工作坊培训的热门课程，更是瑜伽爱好者精进练习的必修课程。本章节在讲解冥想的定义、重要性及注意事项后，为想要精进练习的瑜伽学习者提供了清晰、简洁的双语冥想学习素材。

第六章：课前及课后交流

无论是瑜伽培训课程还是普通会员课程，课前及课后交流都可以拉近老师与学员（或会员）之间的距离，帮助瑜伽老师有的放矢地开展及反思教学活动。因此，本章节涉及师生在课前与课后针对瑜伽学习产生的一般性问答，以新人入馆的视角进行多方面提问，通过瑜伽馆工作人员及老师的回答，消除会员的疑问。

课前交流包括欢迎顾客入馆、了解顾客需求、讲解课程设置、会员卡办理、瑜伽辅具介绍以及课前准备；课后交流包括询问顾客反馈、给出练习建议、提供课后服务及友好道别。

本书还提供了：

1. 注释：对内文带星号的信息均做了相应的解释说明；

2. 梵文词汇简化读音：保留变音符号并引入英文读音方便读者对比学习；

3. 瑜伽体式名称索引表：提供梵文、英文、中文体式名称以及页码，便于读者检索；

4. 梵文词汇表：梳理文中出现的梵文词汇，易于读者随时查阅和识记。

另外，本书配备核心词汇手册——采用日常实例注解正文出现的核心英文词汇；本书底部引用名言出自Swami Satchidananda 的*The Yoga Sutras of Patanjali*（2008）和*To Know Your Self*（2008）两本书，由笔者独立译成中文。

瑜伽英语学习建议：

1. 勤查多练。充分利用网络及语音软件等多渠道确认生词的正确读音，在听清听懂的前提下大胆开口讲。另外，建议读者系统掌握英语音标，培养自学新词汇的能力。

2. 情景记忆。孤立的单词是没有生命力的，一旦你将它放到某一个特定情境中，它便活了起来。在具体的语境下，即便是一词多义的词汇也只能承载单个词义。根据已有例句或者发挥你的想象力和创造力构思新的例句，用一个特定情景将生词牢牢记住。

3. 在做中学。基础知识掌握扎实与否可以在实践中加以检验，通过实践发现自身存在的不足。建议读者在学习本书内容的同时，配合肢体动作以深化对口令的理解与识记，并在实际的运用中一遍遍反思学习。

4. 融会贯通。每学会一个表达时，要认真联想它在哪个体式哪个动作时依然可以用。勤思考、勤对比，相信读者朋友们通过实例学习及亲身实践，定能早日听懂外文瑜伽课程，实现双语瑜伽教学。

【温馨提示】

本书定位为基于瑜伽的英语语言学习教程，文中部分体式未给出相应变体，请务必遵从自己或学员身体的实际情况进行调整。

一个看似简单的瑜伽体式实则包含许多细节，因此不建议瑜伽初学者通过图文或影音资料自学瑜伽，以免造成不必要的伤害。建议在有资质的瑜伽老师的指导下循序渐进地进行练习。

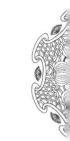

目录

Chapter One
Yoga and You

第一章　瑜伽与你

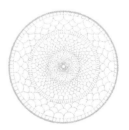

Yoga, as a way of life and a philosophy, can be practiced by anyone with inclination to undertake it, for yoga belongs to humanity as a whole. It is not the property of any one group or any one individual, but can be followed by any and all, in any corner of the globe, regardless of class, creed or religion.

—K. Pattabhi Jois

1.1 About Yoga

1.1.1 Definition and Objectives

The sage Patanjali defined yoga as the restraint of the modifications of the mind-stuff. The word yoga comes from the Sanskrit root "Yuj", meaning "to join, to yoke". It is a series of methods and practices leading to a state of union between individual and universal awareness. In other words, yoga is both union and the way to that union. For the common practitioners' level of understanding, Master Iyengar interpreted yoga as the union of body with the mind and of mind with the soul.

According to *The Yoga Sutras of Patanjali*, the objective of yoga is to weaken what are called the five kleśas (obstacles), i.e., avidyā (ignorance), asmitā (egoism), ragā (attachment), dveṣa (hatred) and abhiniveśa (fear of death). In yoga practice, you can keep experimenting with your body and mind and cultivating your

---

◆ The entire outside world is based on your thoughts and mental attitude. The entire world is your own projection.

瑜伽，作为一种生活方式和哲学，任何有意愿尝试的人都可以练习，因为瑜伽属于整个人类。它不是任何一个团体或任何个人的财产，而是世界任何角落的任何人，不论阶级、信仰或宗教，都可以追随的。

——K. 帕塔比·乔伊斯

1.1 关于瑜伽

1.1.1 定义及目标

Yoga这个词源于梵文词根Yuj，意思是"连接，结合"。它是引领个体意识与普遍意识之间达到联合状态的一系列方法和实践。换句话说，瑜伽既是联合也是实现联合的途径。圣哲帕坦伽利将瑜伽定义为约束心灵的变化。针对普通练习者的理解水平，艾扬格大师将瑜伽解释为身体与心灵、心灵与灵魂的结合。

根据《帕坦伽利的瑜伽经》，瑜伽的目标是削弱所谓的五大障碍（kleśas），即无明（avidyā）、自我（asmitā）、贪恋（ragā）、憎恶（dveṣa）和畏死（abhiniveśa）。在瑜伽习练中，你可以不断地进行身心尝试，通过观察和反思来培养你的觉知。你可以简单地将瑜伽看作一门改善你身心健康的科学，或者是一

◆整个外部世界都基于你的想法和心态。整个世界都是你自己的投射。

awareness through observation and reflection. You might simply consider yoga as a science that improves your physical and mental health or a philosophy that helps liberate your mind from mundane life.

1.1.2 Major Schools of Yoga

Just as there are many paths leading to the top of a mountain, there are different types of yoga for you to choose to find out the truth. These different systems, although practised in various forms, are equally important with a shared goal. Here I will mention a few .

Rāja Yoga

Rāja means king. The word yoga traditionally refers to Rāja Yoga, which is also called Aṣṭāṅga[①] (eight-limbed) Yoga according to *The Yoga Sutras of Patanjali*. The eight limbs of yoga are yama (abstinence), niyama (observance), āsana (posture), prāṇāyāma (regulation of breath), pratyāhāra (sense withdrawal), dhāraṇā (concentration), dhyāna (meditation) and samādhi (super-conscious state).

Haṭha Yoga

Haṭha, which consists of "ha" and "ṭha", refers to the joining of the Sun and the Moon, or the union of the solar and lunar energy. Haṭha Yoga specifically deals with practices for bodily purification which tranquilize the mind and discipline the body. With physical and mental purification and established balance in iḍā and piṅgalā nāḍīs[②], suṣumnā nāḍī opens, enabling the experience of samādhi.

◆ If you can control your mind, you have controlled everything. Then there is nothing in this world to bind you.

门帮助你从世俗生活中解放思想的哲学。

1.1.2 瑜伽的主要流派

正如通往山顶的路有千条万条，为找到真理，你也有很多的瑜伽种类可以选择。尽管这些不同的体系以各种形式习练，但它们是同样重要的而且目标一致。下面我会提到几种。

王瑜伽

Rāja意为"王"。Yoga这个词从传统上来讲指的是王瑜伽。据帕坦伽利的《瑜伽经》，王瑜伽也被称为阿斯汤加（八肢）瑜伽[①]。瑜伽的"八肢"分别是禁制（yama）、劝制（niyama）、体式（āsana）、调息（prāṇāyāma）、制感（pratyāhāra）、专注（dhāraṇā）、冥想（dhyāna）和三摩地（samādhi，超意识状态）。

哈达瑜伽

Haṭha，由"ha"和"ṭha"构成，指的是太阳和月亮的结合，或者阳性能量与阴性能量的联合。哈达瑜伽特别涉及身体净化的练习，这些练习能使心灵平静并磨炼身体。伴随身体和精神的净化以及左脉（iḍā nāḍī）与右脉（piṅgalā nāḍī）[②]之间平衡的建立，中脉（suṣumnā nāḍī）打通，从而开启了三摩地的体验。

◆如果你控制了你的思想，你就控制了一切。那么这个世界上就没有什么可以来缚你了。

Bhakti Yoga

Bhakti Yoga is the yoga of devotion, channeling emotional energy to a higher reality of life. It is generally devotion to God or the supreme consciousness in one of its manifestations. The object of devotion should have strong emotional ties for the devotee, so strong that the devotee's emotional energy is all directed to serving the personal form of the supreme consciousness. When one continually thinks of his object of devotion, one would gradually lose awareness of ego, reduce the kleśas and develop a highly concentrated mind.

Karma Yoga

Karma means action or work, but it's more than this. Karma Yoga is doing work with complete awareness and without agency and attachment to the result. Therefore, it is selfless action that removes impurities of the mind. Activity in Karma Yoga is a sure way to expose one's inner conflicts and personality problems. When one learns how to deal with these problems and stops identifying with one's ego, desires, likes and dislikes will automatically disappear. At that time, one can work with a concentrated mind, fully prepared for meditation and more.

Jñāna Yoga

Jñāna Yoga is yoga of knowledge and wisdom attained through spontaneous self-analysis and investigation of abstract or speculative ideas. There is only one Reality or Truth — ātman or soul independent of body and mind. This ātman is immortal and all-pervading. It is

---

◆ By making the mind clean and pure, you feel you have gone back or you appear to have gone back to your original state.

奉爱瑜伽

Bhakti瑜伽是奉献的瑜伽，它将情感能量引导到更高的生活现实中。它通常是对上帝或最高意识的表现之一做出奉爱。奉献对象对奉献者而言应该有强烈的情感联系，强烈到奉献者的情感能量完全被引导向服务最高意识的人格化身。当一个人不断地念想他的奉献对象时，这个人就会逐渐地失去自我意识，减少障碍，思想变得高度集中。

行动瑜伽

Karma意为行动或工作，但它的意义不止如此。行动瑜伽带着完全的觉知去工作，不带主体意识，不迷恋最终结果。因此，它是能够消除头脑杂质的无私行动。行动瑜伽中的活动一定会暴露一个人的内心冲突和性格问题。当一个人学会如何处理这些问题并不再与自我意识等同起来的时候，欲望、喜好及厌恶将会自动消失。到那个时候，这个人就可以头脑专注地工作，为冥想及更多练习做好充分准备。

智慧瑜伽

Jñāna瑜伽是知识和智慧的瑜伽，这些知识和智慧是通过自发地对抽象或思辨的思想的自我分析和调查而获得的。现实或真理只有一个——ātman或独立于身心的灵魂。这个ātman是不朽的，

◆通过让思想变得干净、纯洁，你会感觉自己已经回到或者看起来好像回到了你最初的状态。

beyond time, space and causation. One will be free and attain self-realization when one identifies with this ātman and gives up thinking of the body and mind.

Kuṇḍalinī Yoga

The word Kuṇḍalinī literally means coiled, coiling (like a serpent). It can be understood as spiritual energy or evolutionary potential that is related to the capacity and awareness of human beings. Kuṇḍalinī Yoga deals with the practical methods that awaken the spiritual force, in the form of a coiled serpent, lying dormant in Mūlādhāra cakra[③] (root cakra). The fundamental aim of Kuṇḍalinī Yoga is to overcome the normal inactivity of higher cakras so that these cakras are stimulated and one is able to experience higher levels of mind.

1.1.3 Yoga and Health

Although yoga is essentially a spiritual science, it contributes a great deal to our physical, emotional and mental health. By regularly practising yoga, our body systems can be balanced and the muscles, tissues, joints and nerves toned, which relax the body, stabilize our emotions and bring mental peace. Here in China, āsana, prāṇāyāma and dhyāna, compared with other limbs of yoga, are more commonly seen in yoga classes and therefore these three limbs will be introduced in detail in the following chapters.

◆ If you detach yourself completely from all the things you have identified yourself with, you realize yourself as the pure "I".

是无所不在的。它超越了时间、空间和因果。当一个人将自身与这一ātman等同起来并放弃对身心的惦念时，这个人将获得自由并达成自我实现。

昆达里尼瑜伽

Kuṇḍalinī这个词的字面意思是盘绕的，（像蛇一样）盘绕。可以将它理解为与人类能力和意识相关的灵性能量或进化潜能。昆达里尼瑜伽涉及唤醒精神的力量的实际方法，这种精神的力量状如一条盘绕的蛇，蛰伏在根轮③（Mūlādhāra cakra）处。昆达里尼瑜伽的基本目标是打破更高层脉轮在常态下的静止状态，这样一来，这些脉轮就会被刺激到，一个人就能够有更高层次的心灵体验。

1.1.3 瑜伽与健康

虽然瑜伽本质上是一门涉及精神层面的科学，但它对我们的身体、情绪和心理健康都有很大帮助。通过规律地练习瑜伽，能够平衡我们的身体系统并强健肌肉、组织、关节和神经，从而放松身体，稳定情绪，带来精神上的平静。在中国，体式、调息和冥想相比于瑜伽的其他"分肢"在瑜伽课上更为常见，因此，下面的章节将详细介绍这"三肢"。

◆如果你将自己从所有你认同的事物中彻底分离出来，你就会意识到自己是那个纯粹的"我"。

1.2 Knowing Your Body

In this part, we will have a general idea of our body, including the major body parts, muscles, bones, joints, internal organs and systems along with common diseases in today's society. Most of the words listed here will be used later in the following chapters. Please read relevant books in anatomy and physiology if you are trying to explore more in yoga therapy.

◆ We should analyze all our motives and try to cultivate selfless thoughts. That is our first and foremost duty.

1.2　了解你的身体

　　在这一部分我们来大致了解一下我们的身体，包括主要身体部位、肌肉、骨、关节、内脏和系统，以及当今社会的常见病。这里列出的大多数词汇在接下来的章节中会用到。如果您想在瑜伽理疗方面有更多的探索，请阅读解剖学和生理学的相关书籍。

◆我们应该分析我们所有的动机并努力培养无私的想法。这是我们的首要职责。

1.2.1 Body Parts

Head and Neck

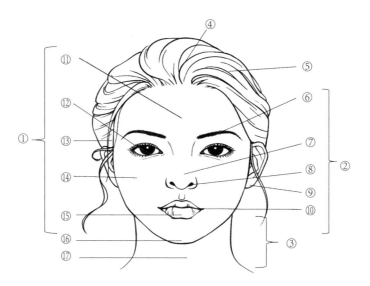

1. **head** [hed]
2. **face** [feɪs]
3. **neck** [nek]
4. **the crown** [kraʊn] **of the head**
5. **hair** [heə]
6. **eyebrow** ['aɪbraʊ]
7. **nose** [nəʊz]
8. **nostril** ['nɒstr(ə)l]
9. **ear** [ɪə]
10. **mouth** [maʊθ]
11. **forehead** ['fɔːhed]
12. **eye** [aɪ]
13. **temple** ['templ]
14. **cheek** [tʃiːk]
15. **lip** [lɪp]
16. **chin** [tʃɪn]
17. **throat** [θrəʊt]
body ['bɒdɪ]
tongue [tʌŋ]
tooth [tuːθ] (*pl.* teeth)

◆ Selfish thoughts will bring misery and selfless ones leave us in peace.

1.2.1　身体部位

头部和颈部

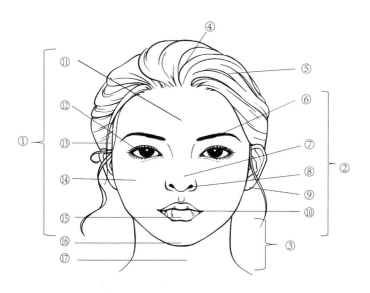

1. 头部	11. 额头
2. 脸	12. 眼睛
3. 颈部	13. 太阳穴
4. 头顶	14. 面颊
5. 头发	15. 唇
6. 眉毛	16. 下巴
7. 鼻子	17. 喉咙
8. 鼻孔	身体
9. 耳朵	舌头
10. 嘴巴	牙齿（复数teeth）

◆自私的想法会带来痛苦，而无私的想法让我们平静。

Torso and Limbs

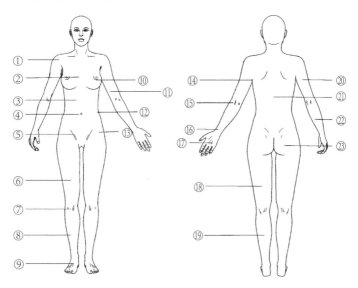

torso ['tɔːsəʊ]

limb [lɪm]

1. shoulder ['ʃəʊldə]

2. chest [tʃest]

3. abdomen ['æbdəmən]

4. navel ['neɪvəl]

5. groin [grɒɪn]

6. leg [leg]

7. knee [niː]

8. shank [ʃæŋk] (or lower leg)

9. foot [fʊt] (*pl.* feet)

10. breast [brest]

11. arm ['aːm]

12. waist [weɪst]

13. hip [hɪp]

14. armpit ['aːmpɪt]

15. elbow ['elbəʊ]

16. wrist [rɪst]

17. hand [hænd]

18. thigh [θaɪ] (or upper leg)

19. calf [kaːf]

20. upper arm ['ʌpə]['aːm]

21. back [bæk]

22. forearm ['fɔːraːm]

23. buttock [bʌtək]

◆ The truth in all scriptures is the same. But the presentation will vary.

躯干和四肢

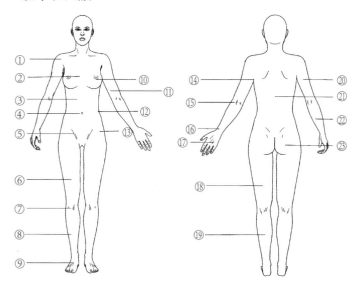

躯干
肢体
1. 肩膀
2. 胸
3. 腹部
4. 肚脐
5. 腹股沟
6. 腿
7. 膝
8. 小腿（或lower leg）
9. 脚（复数feet）
10. 乳房
11. 胳膊

12. 腰
13. 髋，臀
14. 腋窝
15. 肘
16. 手腕
17. 手
18. 大腿（或upper leg）
19. 小腿肚
20. 大臂
21. 背部
22. 小臂
23. 臀部

◆圣经中的真理都是一样的。但展示方式会有所不同。

Hand

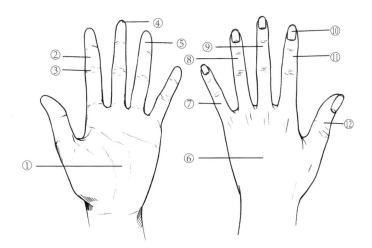

hand [hænd]

1. palm [pɑ:m]

2. finger ['fɪŋgə]

3. knuckle ['nʌkl]

4. fingertip ['fɪŋgətɪp]

5. finger pad ['fɪŋgə][pæd]

6. the back of the hand

7. little finger ['lɪtl]['fɪŋgə]

8. ring finger [rɪŋ]['fɪŋgə]

9. middle finger ['mɪdl]['fɪŋgə]

10. fingernail ['fɪŋgəneɪl]

11. index finger ['ɪndeks]['fɪŋgə]

    (or forefinger ['fɔ:fɪŋgə])

12. thumb [θʌm]

◆ You are going to dispose of all the thoughts as garbage, no doubt, whether they are good or bad, right or wrong, so that the mind will be free from modifications.

手

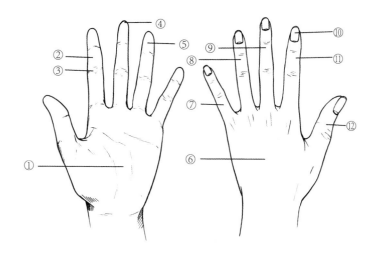

手

1. 手掌

2. 手指

3. 指关节

4. 手指尖

5. 指肚

6. 手背

7. 小指

8. 无名指

9. 中指

10. 手指甲

11. 食指（或forefinger）

12. 大拇指

◆你要把所有的念头都当作垃圾处理掉，毫无疑问，不管它们是好是坏，是对是错，这样心意就会免于波动。

Foot

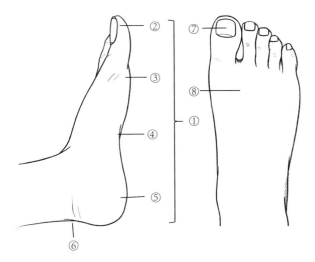

foot [fʊt] (*pl.* feet)

1. sole [səʊl]

2. toe [təʊ]

3. ball (of the foot) [bɔ:l]

4. arch [ɑ:tʃ]

5. heel [hi:l]

6. ankle ['æŋkəl]

7. toenail ['təʊneɪl]

8. instep ['ɪnstep] (or the top of the foot)

Ordinal numbers can be used to describe toes, i.e., big toe (the first toe), the second toe, the third toe, the fourth toe and little toe (the fifth toe).

◆ Don't think that there is no thought in the sleep. If there were no thought and you were completely unconscious, you would not even feel that you had slept.

脚

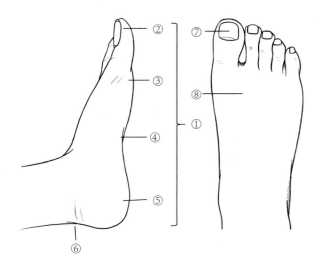

脚（复数feet）

1. 脚掌
2. 脚趾
3. 跖骨球
4. 足弓
5. 脚跟
6. 脚踝
7. 脚指甲
8. 脚背（或the top of the foot）

可以用序数词来描述脚趾，即大脚趾（第一根脚趾），第二根脚趾，第三根脚趾，第四根脚趾和小脚趾（第五根脚趾）。

◆不要以为睡眠中是没有念头的。如果没有念头，并且你完全没有意识，那么你甚至都不会感到自己睡过觉。

1.2.2 Muscles and Skeleton

Muscles

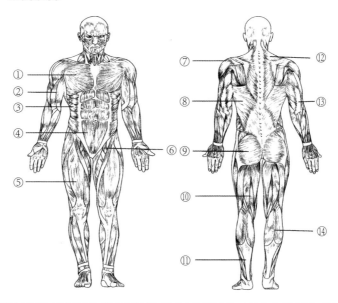

muscle ['mʌsl]
1. pectoralis ['pektərəlɪs]
2. biceps ['baɪseps]
3. intercostal muscles [ˌɪntə'kɒstl] ['mʌslz]
4. abdominal muscles [æb'dɒmɪnəl] ['mʌslz]
5. quadriceps ['kwɒdrɪseps]
6. psoas ['səʊəs]
7. deltoid ['deltɒɪd]

8. latissimus dorsi [lə'tɪsɪməs] ['dɔːsɪ]
9. gluteus maximus ['gluːtɪəs] ['mæksɪməs]
10. hamstring ['hæmstrɪŋ]
11. Achilles tendon [ə'kiliːz] ['tendən]
12. trapezius [trə'piːzɪəs]
13. triceps ['traɪseps]
14. calf muscle [kɑːf]['mʌsl]

◆ It is easy to say, "Control your mind." But, in reality, the mind seems to be controlling us.

1.2.2　肌肉与骨骼

肌肉

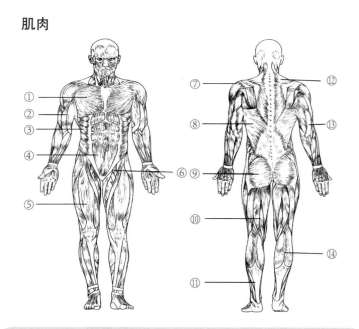

肌肉	8. 背阔肌
1. 胸肌	9. 臀大肌
2. 二头肌	10. 腘绳肌
3. 肋间肌	11. 跟腱
4. 腹肌	12. 斜方肌
5. 四头肌	13. 三头肌
6. 腰肌	14. 腓肠肌
7. 三角肌	

◆说"控制你的心意"很容易。但实际上，心意好像一直在控制我们。

Skeleton

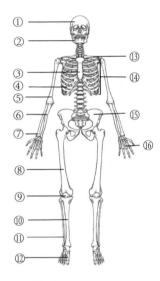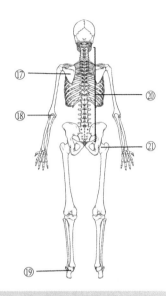

skeleton ['skelɪtn]
1. **skull** [skʌl]
2. **lower jaw** ['ləʊə][dʒɔ:] (or **mandible** ['mændɪbl])
3. **sternum** ['stɜ:nəm]
4. **rib** [rɪb]
5. **humerus** ['hju:mərəs]
6. **ulna** ['ʌlnə]
7. **radius** ['reɪdɪəs]
8. **femur** ['fi:mə]
9. **kneecap** ['ni:kæp] (or **patella** [pə'telə])
10. **shin** [ʃɪn] (or **shinbone** ['ʃɪnbəʊn] / **tibia** ['tɪbɪə])

11. **fibula** ['fɪbjələ]
12. **metatarsal** [ˌmetə'tɑ:sl]
13. **collarbone** ['kɒləbəʊn] (or **clavicle** ['klævɪkl])
14. **ribcage** ['rɪbkeɪdʒ]
15. **pelvis** ['pelvɪs]
16. **metacarpal** [ˌmetə'kɑ:pl]
17. **shoulder blade** ['ʃəʊldə][bleɪd] (or **scapula** ['skæpjələ])
18. **elbow joint** ['elbəʊ][dʒɔɪnt]
19. **ankle joint**
20. **spine** [spaɪn]
21. **hip joint** [hɪp][dʒɔɪnt]

◆ Let us not be like little children who sow a seed today and dig it up tomorrow to see how much the root went down. We need all these three qualities: patience, devotion and faith.

骨骼

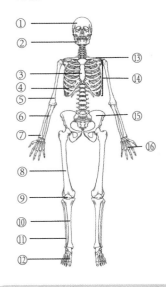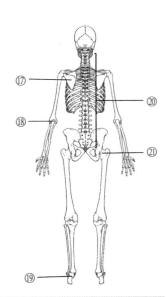

骨骼/骨架	11. 腓骨
1. 颅骨	12. 跖骨
2. 下颌骨（或mandible）	13. 锁骨（或clavicle）
3. 胸骨	14. 胸腔，胸廓
4. 肋骨	15. 骨盆
5. 肱骨	16. 掌骨
6. 尺骨	17. 肩胛骨（或scapula）
7. 桡骨	18. 肘关节
8. 股骨	19. 踝关节
9. 膝盖骨，髌骨（或patella）	20. 脊柱
10. 胫骨，胫（shinbone或tibia）	21. 髋关节

◆我们不要像小孩子一样，今天撒了粒种子明天就挖起来看看根扎得有多深。我们需要这三种品质：耐心，奉献与信念。

Spine

anterior   right lateral   rear
view   view   view

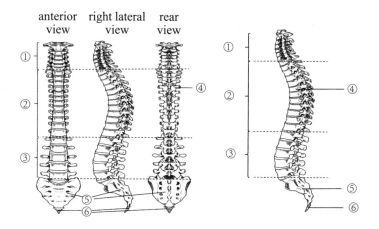

1. **cervical vertebrae** ['sɜːvɪkl]

   ['vɜːtɪbreɪ]

2. **thoracic vertebrae** [θɔːˈræsɪk]

   ['vɜːtɪbreɪ]

3. **lumbar vertebrae** ['lʌmbə]

   ['vɜːtɪbreɪ]

4. **vertebra** ['vɜːtəbrə] (*pl.* vertebrae)

5. **sacrum** ['seɪkrəm]

6. **tailbone** ['teɪlboʊn] (or **coccyx** ['kɒksɪks])

◆ If you are unsettled and anxious to get the result, you are already disturbed; nothing done with that disturbed mind will have quality.

脊柱

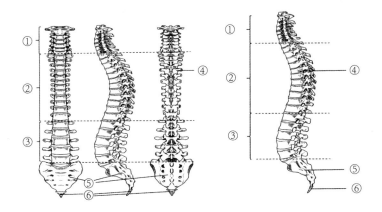

1. 颈椎
2. 胸椎
3. 腰椎

4. 椎骨（复数vertebrae）
5. 骶骨
6. 尾骨，尾椎（或coccyx）

◆如果你心绪不宁，急于得到结果，那你已经受到干扰了；心神不安做任何事都没有质量可言。

1.2.3 Internal Organs and Systems

Internal Organs

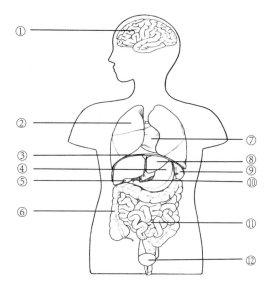

internal organ [ɪn'tɜ:nl]['ɔ:gən]   7. heart [hɑ:t]

1. brain [breɪn]   8. liver ['lɪvə]

2. lung [lʌŋ]   9. spleen [spli:n]

3. diaphragm ['daɪəfræm]   10. pancreas ['pæŋkrɪəs]

4. stomach ['stʌmək]   11. small intestine [smɔ:l][ɪn'testɪn]

5. gall bladder ['gɔ:l][blædə]   12. bladder ['blædə]

6. large intestine [lɑ:dʒ][ɪn'testɪn]

◆ Every desire brings its own color to the mind. The moment you color the mind, a ripple is formed, just as when a stone is thrown into a calm lake it creates waves in the water.

1.2.3　内脏器官和系统

内脏器官

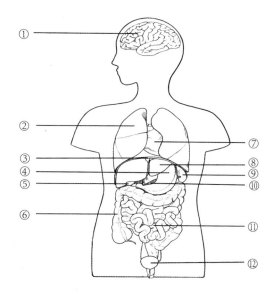

内脏/内脏器官	7. 心脏
1. 大脑	8. 肝脏
2. 肺	9. 脾
3. 横膈膜	10. 胰腺
4. 胃	11. 小肠
5. 胆囊	12. 膀胱
6. 大肠	

◆每种欲望都会给心灵带来自己的色彩。当你给心灵涂上色彩的那一刻，就会产生一道涟漪，就像把一块石头扔进平静的湖中，它会在水中激起水波一样。

System

The organs of the body work together in systems.

integumentary systems [ɪn,tegjʊ'mentərɪ]['sɪstəmz]

The integumentary systems include the skin and accessory organs, such as the hair, nails, sweat glands and so on. The skin protects underlying tissues and can help regulate body temperature.

skeletal systems ['skelətəl]['sɪstəmz]

muscular systems ['mʌskjələ]['sɪstəmz]

The skeletal systems and muscular systems together offer the body support and enable the body and its parts to move.

nervous systems ['nɜ:vəs]['sɪstəmz]

endocrine systems ['endəʊkraɪn]['sɪstəmz]

The nervous systems consist of the brain, spinal cord and associated nerves while the endocrine systems largely consist of the hormonal glands. These two systems help maintain a relatively constant internal environment by coordinating and regulating the functions of the body's other systems.

respiratory systems [rə'spɪrətrɪ]['sɪstəmz]

The respiratory systems consist of the lungs and the respiratory tract that brings oxygen into the lungs and takes carbon dioxide out of the lungs.

cardiovascular systems [ˌkɑ:dɪəʊ'væskjələ]['sɪstəmz]

The cardiovascular systems consist of the heart and the blood vessels that carry blood through the body.

lymphatic systems [lɪm'fætɪk]['sɪstəmz]

Blood contains cells produced by the lymphatic systems, which

---

◆ When you want to do something constantly, your mind should not be distracted by other desires.

系统

身体的各个器官在系统中协同运作。

皮肤系统

皮肤系统包括皮肤和附属器官，如头发、指甲、汗腺等。皮肤保护皮下组织并能够帮助调节体温。

骨骼系统

肌肉系统

骨骼系统和肌肉系统共同为身体提供支撑，使身体的每个部分能够动起来。

神经系统

内分泌系统

神经系统由大脑、脊髓和相关神经组成，而内分泌系统主要由内分泌腺组成。这两个系统通过协调和调节身体其他系统的功能，来帮助维持一个相对恒定的内部环境。

呼吸系统

呼吸系统由肺和呼吸道组成，呼吸道将氧气带入肺部并将二氧化碳带出肺部。

心血管系统

心血管系统由心脏和在体内输送血液的血管组成。

淋巴系统

血液里含有淋巴系统产生的细胞，淋巴系统可以保护身体免

◆当你想持续做某件事情时，你的精力不应该被其他欲望分散。

protect the body from diseases.

digestive systems [daɪ'dʒestɪv]['sɪstəmz]

The digestive systems consist of the mouth, esophagus, stomach, small intestines and large intestines together with the accessory organs.

urinary systems ['jʊərɪnərɪ]['sɪstəmz]

The urinary systems mainly include the kidneys and the urinary bladder.

reproductive systems [ˌriːprə'dʌktɪv]['sɪstəmz]

The male and female reproductive systems are different. The male reproductive systems include the penis, testes and other glands while the female reproductive systems include ovaries, uterine tubes, uterus, vagina and external genitalia.

1.2.4 Common Diseases

acidity [ə'sɪdətɪ]

arthritis [ɑː'θraɪtɪs]

asthma ['æsmə]

backache ['bækeɪk]

breathlessness ['breθləsnəs]

bronchitis [brɒŋ'kaɪtɪs]

cancer ['kænsə]

cold [kəʊld]

coronary artery diseases (CAD) ['kɒrənrɪ]['ɑːtərɪ][dɪ'zɪzɪs]

◆ In fact, you need not even practise meditation if your mind is completely free from all selfish desires.

受疾病侵扰。

消化系统

消化系统包括口、食道、胃、小肠、大肠及附属器官。

泌尿系统

泌尿系统主要包括肾脏和膀胱。

生殖系统

男性和女性的生殖系统不同。男性生殖系统包括阴茎、睾丸和其他腺体，而女性生殖系统包括卵巢、输卵管、子宫、阴道和外生殖器。

1.2.4 常见疾病

胃酸过多

关节炎

哮喘

背部疼痛

呼吸急促，气喘

支气管炎

癌症

感冒

冠状动脉疾病，冠心病

◆事实上，如果你的心意完全摆脱了所有自私的欲望，你甚至不需要练习冥想。

constipation [ˌkɒnstɪˈpeɪʃn]

depression [dɪˈpreʃn]

diabetes [ˌdaɪəˈbiːtiːz]

diarrhea [ˌdaɪəˈrɪə]

dizziness [ˈdɪzɪnəs]

duodenal ulcers [ˌdjuːəˈdiːnl][ˈʌlsəz]

fever [ˈfiːvə]

flatulence [ˈflætjʊləns]

flu [fluː]

gastritis [gæˈstraɪtɪs]

gastrointestinal ulcer [ˌgæstrəʊɪnˈtestɪnl][ˈʌlsə]

headache [ˈhedeɪk]

heartburn [ˈhɑːtbɜːn]

heart disease [hɑːt][dɪˈziːz]

heart problem [hɑːt][ˈprɒbləm]

hernia [ˈhɜːnɪə]

herniated cervical disc [ˈhɜːnɪeɪtɪd][ˈsɜːvɪkl][dɪsk]

herniated/slipped disc [ˈhɜːnɪeɪtɪd] / [slɪpt][dɪsk]

high blood pressure [haɪ][blʌd][ˈpreʃə]

hunchback [ˈhʌntʃbæk]

indigestion [ˌɪndɪˈdʒestʃən]

◆ When we say unattached, it means without personal desires. If you really want to be greedy, be greedy in serving others.

便秘

抑郁，抑郁症

糖尿病

腹泻，痢疾

头晕

十二指肠溃疡

发热，发烧

胀气

流感

胃炎

消化道溃疡

头痛

胃灼热，烧心

心脏病

心脏问题

疝气

颈椎间盘突出症

椎间盘突出

高血压

驼背

消化不良

◆当我们说不依恋时，意思是没有个人欲望。如果你真的想要贪婪，那就贪婪地服务他人。

inflammation [ˌɪnfləˈmeɪʃn]

insomnia [ɪnˈsɒmnɪə]

intestinal tuberculosis [ɪnˈtestɪnl][tjuːˌbɜːkjuˈləʊsɪs]

irregular periods [ɪˈreɡjələ][pɪərɪədz]

ischial bursitis [ˈɪskɪəl][ˌbɜːˈsaɪtɪs]

knee injury [niː][ˈɪndʒərɪ]

low blood pressure [ləʊ][blʌd][ˈpreʃə]

lumbago [lʌmˈbeɪɡəʊ]

lumbar disc herniation [ˈlʌmbə][dɪsk][ˌhɜːnɪˈeɪʃən]

lumbar lordosis [ˈlʌmbə][lɔːˈdəʊsɪs]

meniscal tears [ˈmənɪskl][tɪəz]

menstrual cramps [ˈmenstruəl][kræmps]

menstrual discomfort [ˈmenstruəl][dɪsˈkʌmfət]

menstrual disorders [ˈmenstruəl][dɪsˈɔːdəz]

nausea [ˈnɔːzɪə]

osteoporosis [ˌɒstɪəʊpəˈrəʊsɪs]

palpitation [pælpɪˈteɪʃən]

Parkinson's disease [ˈpaːkɪnsənz][dɪˈziːz]

peptic ulcer [ˈpeptɪk][ˈʌlsə]

rash [ræʃ]

respiratory ailment [rəˈspɪrətrɪ][ˈeɪlmənt]

◆ The selfless person is the most selfish one. Why? Because a selfless person doesn't want to lose his or her peace and happiness.

发炎，炎症

失眠

肠结核

月经不规律

坐骨滑囊炎

膝关节损伤

低血压

腰痛

腰椎间盘突出症

腰椎前凸

半月板撕裂

经期痉挛，痛经

经期不适

月经失调，经期紊乱

恶心

骨质疏松症

心悸

帕金森病

消化性溃疡

皮疹

呼吸系统疾病

◆无私的人是最自私的人。为什么？因为一个无私的人不想失去他或她的平静与幸福。

rheumatism ['ruːmətɪzəm]

rickets ['rɪkɪts]

sciatica [saɪ'ætɪkə]

scoliosis [ˌskəʊlɪ'əʊsɪs]

shoulder and neck problems

spine injury [spaɪn]['ɪndʒərɪ]

stomachache ['stʌməkeɪk]

stroke [strəʊk]

trochanteric bursitis [trəʊtʃæn'tərɪk][ˌbɜː'saɪtɪs]

urinary system disorder ['jʊərɪnərɪ]['sɪstəm][dɪs'ɔːdə]

weak heart [wiːk][hɑːt]

◆ Every desire binds you and brings restlessness. To be liberated, you have to be completely desireless.

风湿病

佝偻病

坐骨神经痛

脊柱侧凸，脊柱侧弯

肩颈问题

脊柱损伤

胃痛，腹痛

中风

大粗隆滑囊炎

泌尿系统紊乱

心脏衰弱

◆每一种欲望都会束缚你，带来不安。要获得解放，你必须完全没有欲望。

Chapter Two
Yogāsanas

第二章 瑜伽体式

Yoga is a fine art and seeks to express the artist's abilities to the fullest possible extent. While most artists need an instrument, such as a paintbrush or a violin, to express their art, the only instruments a yogi needs are his body and his mind.

—B.K.S Iyengar

2.1 Standing Poses

2.1.1 Tāḍāsana / Mountain pose

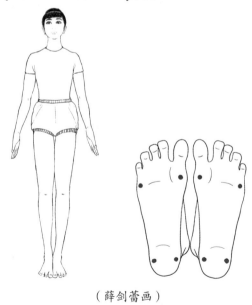

（薛剑蕾画）

◆ Is it possible to be desireless? No. But any desires without a personal or selfish motive will never bind you.

　　瑜伽是一门精妙的艺术，它力求最大程度地表达艺术家的能力。虽然大多数艺术家需要一种工具，如画笔或小提琴，来表达他们的艺术，但瑜伽修行者唯一需要的工具是他自己的身体和思想。

——B.K.S 艾扬格

2.1　站立体式

2.1.1　山式

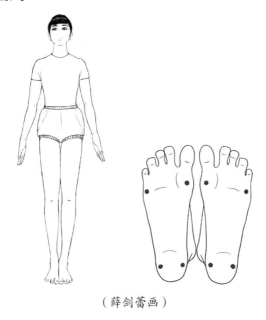

（薛剑蕾画）

　　◆没有欲望可能吗？不可能。但是任何没有个人或自私动机的欲望永远都不会来缚你。

Step-by-step Instructions

Feet together, toes, ankles and heels touching, or stand with your feet parallel and hip-width apart.

Lift and spread your toes as you press all four corners of each foot into the ground, anchoring the base of your big toes.

See that your body weight is spread evenly over your feet.

Activate your legs by engaging your thigh muscles and lifting your kneecaps. Tuck your tailbone in and make sure that your pelvis is parallel to the ground.

Lift your spine and keep it perpendicular to the floor. Draw your lower ribs gently in, aligning your ribcage over your pelvis.

Relax your shoulders away from your ears, widening them horizontally to create space between your shoulder blades and across your chest.

Extend your arms along the sides of your body, with your palms facing your thighs and fingers pointing down.

Draw your chin slightly back and in, keeping your head and spine in a straight line, with your gaze resting on the horizon.

Breathe normally during all the steps of this pose. Hold this pose for 20 to 30 seconds.

Benefits

Mountain pose can help
  · improve posture
  · strengthen the thighs, knees and ankles
  · tone the buttock muscles

◆ There is joy in losing everything, and in giving everything. You cannot be eternally happy by possessing things.

步骤说明

双脚并拢，脚趾、脚踝及脚跟相触，或者双脚平行站立，打开与髋同宽。

每只脚的四个角都下压地面的同时，脚趾提起并分开，大脚趾底部稳固。

确保身体重量均匀地分布在双脚上。

通过启动大腿肌肉和髌骨上提激活双腿。尾骨内收并确保骨盆平行于地面。

脊柱上提，并保持垂直于地面。肋骨下端轻柔地向内收，胸腔处于骨盆正上方。

双肩放松远离双耳，水平方向展开，在肩胛骨之间及整个胸部区域创造空间。

手臂沿身体两侧伸展，掌心朝向大腿，手指朝下。

下巴微微向后内收，头部与脊柱保持在一条直线上，目光凝视地平线。

在该体式的所有步骤中正常呼吸。保持这个体式20到30秒。

益处

山式能够帮助

· 改善体态

· 强健大腿、双膝及脚踝

· 强健臀部肌肉

◆失去一切和给予一切都蕴含快乐。你不可能通过拥有物件而永久幸福。

Contraindications and Cautions

People with Parkinson's disease or a disc problem may stand facing a wall with palms placed on it. Those that have scoliosis should rest the spine against the protruding edge of two adjoining walls.

Words and Expressions / 词汇表达

mountain ['maʊntən] *n.* 高山，山岳　*e.g.* to climb a mountain 爬山

pose [pəʊz] *n.* 姿势，姿态　*e.g.* yoga pose 瑜伽姿势，瑜伽体式

step-by-step ['step-baɪ-'step] *adj.* 循序渐进的　*e.g.* step-by-step guidance 循序渐进的指导

instruction [ɪn'strʌkʃn] *n.* 指令，教导　*e.g.* verbal instruction 口头指令

together [tə'geðə(r)] *adv.* 一起　*e.g.* put together 放在一起

touch [tʌtʃ] *v.* 接触，触碰　*e.g.* touch your face 触碰你的脸

stand [stænd] *v.* 站立　*e.g.* stand up 站起来

with [wɪð] *prep.* 伴随　*e.g.* rest with eyes closed 闭眼休息 / *prep.* 有　*e.g.* a girl with short hair 一个短发女孩

parallel ['pærəlel] *adj.* 平行的　*e.g.* parallel line 平行线

width [wɪdθ] *n.* 宽度　*e.g.* the width of... ······的宽度

apart [ə'pɑːt] *adv.* 相距，分开　*e.g.* tell apart 区别，分辨

lift [lɪft] *v.* 举起，抬起　*e.g.* lift up 举起

spread [spred] *v.* 展开，伸展　*e.g.* spread your legs 双腿分开 / *v.* 使分散，使分布　*e.g.* spread risk 分散风险

◆ By renouncing worldly things, you possess the most important sacred property: your peace.

禁忌和注意事项

患有帕金森病或椎间盘有问题的人可以面朝墙壁站立，手掌放在墙上。脊柱侧弯者应将脊柱靠在相邻两面墙的突出边缘上。

press [pres] *v.* 压，按　***e.g.*** press the red button 按红色的按钮
press...into... 压入

all [ɔːl] *adj.* 全部的，所有的　***e.g.*** sit up all night 彻夜不眠

corner ['kɔːnə] *n.* 角　***e.g.*** in the corner 在角落里

earth [ɜːθ] *n.* 土地，陆地　***e.g.*** the ends of the earth 天涯海角

anchor ['æŋkə(r)] *v.* 使固定　***e.g.*** anchor a plant in flowerpot 把植物固定在花盆里

base [beɪs] *n.* 基底，底面，底部　***e.g.*** the base of the spine 脊柱末端

see that... 注意，务必，确保

weight [weɪt] *n.* 重量　***e.g.*** body weight 体重

evenly ['iːvnlɪ] *adv.* 均匀地，平等地　***e.g.*** evenly distributed 均匀分布

over ['əʊvə] *prep.* 在……上面　***e.g.*** arms over your head 手臂举过头顶

activate ['æktɪveɪt] *v.* 刺激，激活　***e.g.*** activate your core muscles 激活你的核心肌肉

by [baɪ] *prep.* 通过，由　***e.g.*** by air 通过航空途径，乘飞机

engage [ɪn'geɪdʒ] *v.* 使用，占用　***e.g.*** engage your core muscles 调动

◆通过放弃世俗的东西，你拥有了最重要的神圣财产：你的平静。

46　An Introductory Guidebook of Yoga English
Chapter Two

身体核心肌肉

tuck [tʌk] *v.* 卷起，收拢　*e.g.* tuck your hair under your cap 把头发拢起来塞进帽子里

in [ɪn] *adv.* 朝里，在里面　*e.g.* come in 进入

make sure (that) 确保

(be) parallel to 平行于

ground [graʊnd] *n.* 地面，土地　*e.g.* sit on the ground 坐在地上

keep [kiːp] *v.* 保持　*e.g.* keep healthy 保持健康

perpendicular to 垂直于

floor [flɔː] *n.* 地板，地面　*e.g.* sit on the floor 坐在地板上

draw [drɔː] *v.* 拉，牵引　*e.g.* draw your belly in 腹部内收

lower ['ləʊə] *adj.* 下方的，下面的　*e.g.* lower lip 下嘴唇

gently ['dʒentlɪ] *adv.* 轻轻地，温和地　*e.g.* gently bend backward 轻柔地后弯

align [ə'laɪn] *v.* 对齐，对准　*e.g.* align camera 对齐摄像机

relax [rɪ'læks] *v.* 放松，使松弛　*e.g.* relax your shoulders 放松肩膀

away from 远离，离开

widen ['waɪdn] *v.* 变宽，扩大　*e.g.* widen the gap 拉大差距

horizontally [ˌhɒrɪ'zɒntəlɪ] *adv.* 水平地　*e.g.* walk horizontally 横着走

to [tuː] *prep.*（用于表示动作的动词之后）为了给，以提供　*e.g.* come to help 过来帮忙 / *prep.*（表示范围或一段时间的结尾或界限）到，至　*e.g.* a drop in profits from 5 million to 1 million 利润从500万降至100万

create [kri'eɪt] *v.* 创造　*e.g.* create new opportunities 创造新的机会

◆ If our minds are free from selfishness and there is sacrifice in everyone's lives, the very world will become a heaven, an abode of peace and bliss.

space [speɪs] *n.* 空间　***e.g.*** living space 生存空间

between [bɪ'twiːn] *prep.* 在……之间　***e.g.*** between us 在我们之间

across [ə'krɒs] *prep.* 在（身体某部位）上　***e.g.*** hit somebody across the face 打某人的脸

extend [ɪk'stend] *v.* 延伸，伸展　***e.g.*** extend your arms 伸展你的手臂

along [ə'lɒŋ] *prep.* 沿着，顺着　***e.g.*** walk along this road 沿这条路走

side [saɪd] *n.* 侧面，旁边　***e.g.*** left side 左侧

face [feɪs] *v.* 面向，朝向　***e.g.*** face up 脸朝上

point [pɔɪnt] *v.* 指向，朝向　***e.g.*** point in the wrong direction 指向错误的方向

down [daʊn] *adv.* 向下，在下面　***e.g.*** sit down 坐下

slightly ['slaɪtlɪ] *adv.* 稍微地，轻微地　***e.g.*** slightly different 略有不同

back [bæk] *adv.* 向后地　***e.g.*** step back 退一步

in a straight line 在一条直线上

gaze [geɪz] *n.* 凝视，注视　***e.g.*** close gaze 密切注视

rest on 停留在，被搁在

horizon [hə'raɪzn] *n.* 地平线，视野　***e.g.*** on the horizon 在地平线上

breathe [briːð] *v.* 呼吸　***e.g.*** breathe in 吸气

normally ['nɔːməlɪ] *adv.* 正常地，通常地　***e.g.*** breathe normally 正常地呼吸

during ['djʊərɪŋ] *prep.* 在……的期间　***e.g.*** during the day 在白天

step [step] *n.* 步，步骤　***e.g.*** the first step 第一步

hold [həʊld] *v.* 使保持（在某位置）　***e.g.*** hold this posture 保持这个姿势

◆如果我们的思想不再自私，每个人在生活中都作出些牺牲，那么这个世界就会变成天堂，一个安宁喜乐的住所。

for [fɔ:] *prep.*（表示一段时间） *e.g.* for now 目前

second ['sekənd] 秒 *e.g.* a few seconds 几秒钟

benefit ['benɪfɪt] *n.* 利益，益处 *e.g.* be of benefit to... 对……有好处

help [help] *v.* 帮助 *e.g.* May I help you? 我能为您做点什么吗?

improve [ɪm'pru:v] *v.* 改善，提高，增进 *e.g.* improve memory 增强记忆力

posture ['pɒstʃə] *n.* 姿势，身姿 *e.g.* sitting posture 坐姿

strengthen ['streŋθn] *v.* 增强，加强 *e.g.* strengthen environmental protection 增强环境保护

tone [təʊn] *v.* 使强健，使健壮 *e.g.* tone your limbs 强健四肢

contraindication [ˌkɒntrəˌɪndɪ'keɪʃn] *n.* 禁忌证 *e.g.* dietetic contraindication 饮食禁忌

◆ What is due to us will come. We don't need to worry about it.

caution ['kɔːʃn] *n.*（对危险或风险的）警告，告诫　***e.g.*** a word of caution 一句警告

problem ['prɒbləm] *n.* 问题，难题　***e.g.*** social problem 社会问题

place...on... 把……放在……上

rest...against...（使）靠在……上

protruding [prə'truːdɪŋ] *adj.* 突出的，伸出的　***e.g.*** protruding abdomen 凸出的腹部

edge [edʒ] *n.* 边缘　***e.g.*** outer edge 外缘

adjoining [ə'dʒɔɪnɪŋ] *adj.* 邻接的，毗邻的　***e.g.*** an adjoining room 隔壁房间

wall [wɔːl] *n.* 墙　***e.g.*** a white wall 一堵白墙

◆该是我们得的，无需担心便会得到。

2.1.2   Utkaṭāsana / Chair pose

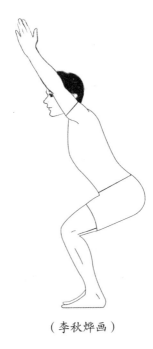

(李秋烨画)

Step-by-step Instructions

Stand in Mountain pose. Inhale, extend your arms overhead with elbows straight or stretch your arms out in front of your body to shoulder height.

Exhale, bend your knees, lower your hips down and try to bring your thighs parallel to the floor, pressing your heels into the floor. Be careful not to extend your knees beyond the toes.

Tuck your tailbone in, stretch your torso upward and keep your chest lifted.

◆ We will never be afraid of the world if we learn how to enjoy it.

2.1.2 幻椅式

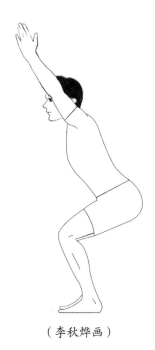

（李秋烨画）

步骤说明

山式站立。吸气，双臂伸展过头顶，手肘伸直，或双臂体前伸展，与肩同高。

呼气，屈双膝，沉髋向下，尽量让大腿与地板平行，脚跟下压地板。注意膝盖不要超过脚趾。

尾骨内收，躯干伸展向上，保持胸腔上提。

◆如果我们学会如何享受这个世界，就永远都不会害怕它。

Hold this pose for 20 to 30 seconds, breathing normally.

Inhale, straighten your legs. Exhale, release your arms to your sides into Mountain pose.

Benefits

Chair pose can help
- remove stiffness in the shoulders and stretch the chest
- strengthen the ankles, thighs, calves and spine
- stimulate the abdominal organs, diaphragm and heart

Contraindications and Cautions

Be careful with this pose if you have headache, insomnia and low blood pressure.

Words and Expressions / 词汇表达

chair [tʃeə] *n.* 椅子　*e.g.* a chair 一把椅子

in [ɪn] *prep.* 以……方式　*e.g.* pay in cash 用现金支付 / *prep.* 在（某范围或空间内的）某一处　*e.g.* in the heart chakra 在心轮处

inhale [ɪn'heɪl] *v.* 吸气　*e.g.* inhale deeply 深深地吸气

overhead [əʊvə'hed] *adv.* 在头顶上方　*e.g.* fly overhead 飞过头顶

straight [streɪt] *adj.* 直的，笔直的　*e.g.* a straight road 一条笔直的路

stretch out 伸出

in front of 在……前面

height [haɪt] *n.* 高度　*e.g.* maximum height 最大高度

◆ A focused mind gains power, and when that powerful mind concentrates on an object, the entire knowledge of that object is revealed to it.

保持这个体式20到30秒，正常呼吸。

吸气，双腿伸直。呼气，双臂落回到身体两侧进入山式。

益处

幻椅式能够帮助

· 消除肩膀僵硬感，扩展胸部

· 强健脚踝、大腿、小腿肚和脊柱

· 刺激腹内器官、横膈膜及心脏

禁忌和注意事项

如果你有头痛、失眠及低血压，则应谨慎练习该体式。

exhale [eks'heɪl] *v.* 呼气　***e.g.*** slowly exhale 慢慢地呼气

bend [bend] *v.* 弯曲，折弯　***e.g.*** bend your elbows 屈肘

lower ['ləʊə] *v.* 放下，降低　***e.g.*** lower one's head 低下头

try to 试着，努力，设法

bring [brɪŋ] *v.* 使朝（某方向或按某方式）移动　***e.g.*** bring your hands to the front of your chest 双手来到胸前

beyond [bɪ'jɒnd] *prep.* 超过，越过　***e.g.*** extend beyond... 延伸到……之外

be careful (not) to 小心（不要）

◆专注的心意会获得力量，当这个强大的心意专注于一个对象时，关于这个对象的全部知识就会显现给它。

stretch [stretʃ] *v.* 伸展，拉伸　*e.g.* stretch the chest 伸展胸腔

upward [ˈʌpwəd] *adv.* 向上地　*e.g.* climb upward 向上爬

straighten [ˈstreɪtn] *v.* 使拉直，挺直　*e.g.* straighten both legs 伸直双腿

release [rɪˈliːs] *v.* 放开，松开　*e.g.* release your hands 松开双手

to [tuː] *prep.* 到达（某处）　*e.g.* walk to the left 走到左边

into [ˈɪntuː] *prep.* 进入　*e.g.* jump into the air 跳起来

remove [rɪˈmuːv] *v.* 使消失　*e.g.* remove obstacles 排除障碍

2.1.3　Utthita Trikoṇāsana / Extended Triangle pose[④]

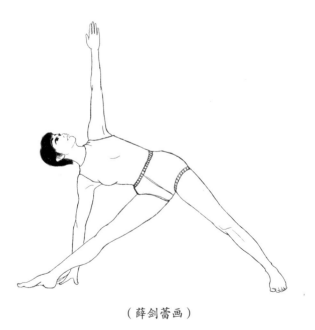

（薛剑蕾画）

◆ The mind can't function on the same level always — it has its heights and depths.

stiffness ['stɪfnəs] *n.* 僵硬　　***e.g.*** remove stiffness 消除僵硬感

stimulate ['stɪmjuleɪt] *v.* 刺激，促进　　***e.g.*** stimulate the ovaries 促进卵巢功能

abdominal [æb'dɒmɪnəl] *adj.* 腹部的　　***e.g.*** abdominal muscles 腹肌

be careful with 对……小心，警惕

2.1.3　三角伸展式④

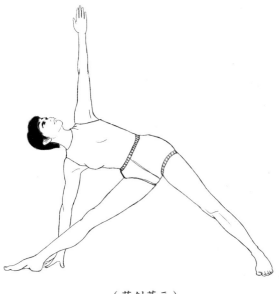

（薛剑蕾画）

◆头脑不能总是在同一水平上运作——它有它的高度和深度。

Step-by-step Instructions

Start in Mountain pose. Walk or jump your feet 1~1.2 metres (3.5 to 4 feet) apart. Turn the right foot out 90 degrees and the left slightly in.

Lift your toes and ground all four corners of both feet evenly, using your back heel as an anchor for the pose.

Inhale, lift your arms laterally to shoulder height.

Exhale, keeping the sides of your torso even, extend your right arm out over your right leg, parallel to the earth. Rest your right hand on the floor outside your right foot (If you have difficulty doing so, try to rest your right hand on the shin, ankle or a yoga block near your ankle).

Turn your pelvis, abdomen and chest toward the ceiling using the pushing force of your right hand. Tuck your shoulder blades in and open your chest.

Make sure that your left arm stretched straight up in line with your right arm, perpendicular to the floor.

Keep both sides of your neck evenly long and your head in a straight line with the spine. Turn your head and look up.

Hold this pose for 20 to 30 seconds with normal breathing.

As you inhale, come up, reverse your feet and repeat on the other side for the same length of time.

Benefits

Extended Triangle pose can help
 · stretch and strengthen the thighs, knees and ankles

◆ Remember, yoga practice is like an obstacle race; many obstructions are purposely put on the way for us to pass through.

步骤说明

由山式开始。走或跳开1到1.2米（3.5到4英尺）的距离。右脚向外打开90度，左脚稍向内收。

脚趾上提，双脚上四个角均匀落地，用后脚脚跟当作体式的固定点。

吸气，手臂从体侧向上抬起，与肩同高。

呼气，保持躯干两侧等长，右臂于右腿上方向外伸展，与地面平行。右手放在右脚外侧的地板上（如果这样做有困难，尝试将右手放在小腿胫骨、脚踝或者靠近脚踝的瑜伽砖上）。

借助右手的推力，转动骨盆、腹部和胸腔朝向天花板。肩胛骨内收，打开胸腔。

确保左臂伸直向上与右臂在一条直线上，垂直于地板。

保持颈部两侧等长，头与脊柱在一条直线上。转动头部向上看。

保持这个体式20到30秒，正常呼吸。

随着吸气，起身，反转脚的位置，换另一侧重复练习，保持相同时长。

益处

三角伸展式可以帮助

·拉伸及强健大腿、双膝和脚踝

◆记住，瑜伽练习就像障碍赛跑；许多障碍物是故意放在路上让我们通过的。

· relieve gastritis, indigestion, acidity, flatulence and backache

· stimulate the abdominal organs

Contraindications and Cautions

Be careful with this pose if you have diarrhea, headache and low blood pressure. If you have heart disease, practise against a wall and keep the top arm on the hip. If you have high blood pressure, look down at the floor in the final pose. If you have neck problems, you can look straight ahead to make it easier on the neck.

Words and Expressions / 词汇表达

extended [ɪk'stendɪd] *adj.* 延长的，扩展的   *e.g.* extended family（几代同堂的）大家庭

triangle ['traɪæŋgl] *adj.* 三角（形）   *e.g.* triangle trade 三角贸易

start [stɑːt] *v.* 开始   *e.g.* start to do something 开始做某事

walk [wɔːk] *v.* 走，走过   *e.g.* walk away 走开

jump [dʒʌmp] *v.* 跳跃   *e.g.* jump up 跳起来

metre ['miːtə] *n.* 米（美式英语记作meter，缩写为m）   *e.g.* square metre 平方米

foot [fʊt] *n.* 英尺   *e.g.* Foot is a unit for measuring length. 英尺是一个长度测量单位。

turn [tɜːn] *v.* 转动，转向   *e.g.* turn around 转身

right [raɪt] *adj.* 右边的   *e.g.* right hand 右手

out [aʊt] *adv.* 向外   *e.g.* breathe out 呼气

◆ When you decide on one thing, stick to it whatever happens. There's no value in digging shallow wells in a hundred places. Decide on one place and dig deep.

·缓解胃炎、消化不良、胃酸、胀气及背部疼痛

·刺激腹内器官

禁忌和注意事项

如果你有腹泻、头痛和低血压，请谨慎练习该体式。如果你有心脏病，靠墙练习并将上方手放在髋部。如果有高血压，在终极体式时向下看向地板。如果颈部有问题，可以直视前方让颈部更轻松一点。

degree [dɪ'griː] *n.*（指角度、经纬度）度　*e.g.* an angle of 5 degrees 5 度角

left [left] *adj.* 左边的　*e.g.* left foot 左脚

ground [graʊnd] *v.* 使接触地面　*e.g.* ground your sitting bones 坐骨落地

use [juːz] *v.* 使用　*e.g.* use props 使用辅具

back [bæk] *adj.* 后面的　*e.g.* back door 后门

as [æz] *prep.* 作为，当作　*e.g.* work as 充当，作为　use...as... 把……当作……使用

anchor ['æŋkə] *n.* 可靠或主要的支撑　*e.g.* anchor point 固定点

for [fɔː] *prep.* 以帮助，为了　*e.g.* do something for you 为你而做

laterally ['lætərəlɪ] *adv.* 旁边地　*e.g.* bend laterally 侧弯

even ['iːvn] *adj.* 均衡的，相等的　*e.g.* even spacing 间隔匀称

◆当你决定做一件事，不管发生什么，都要坚持下去。在一百个地方挖浅井没有任何价值。选定一个地方，深入挖掘。

extend out 伸出，伸展

rest [rest] *v.* 使倚靠，使停放   *e.g.* rest... on... 使……停放在……上

on [ɒn] *prep.* 在……上   *e.g.* sit on the floor 坐在地板上 / *prep.*（与某些名词连用，表示影响到） *e.g.* a ban on smoking 对吸烟的禁令

outside [ˌaʊt'saɪd] *prep.* 在……外面   *e.g.* outside the classroom 在教室外

have difficulty (in) doing something 做……有困难

so [səʊ] *adv.* 如此（用以指代刚刚提及的事） *e.g.* if so 如果是这样的话

toward [tə'wɔːd] *prep.*（同 towards）朝向   *e.g.* walk toward 走向

ceiling ['siːlɪŋ] *n.* 天花板   *e.g.* glass ceiling 玻璃天花板

pushing force 推力

straight [streɪt] *adv.* 直地，径直地   *e.g.* look straight at 直视

up [ʌp] *adv.* 向上   *e.g.* stand up 站起来

in line with 在一条直线上

long [lɒŋ] *adj.* 长的   *e.g.* long hair 长发

look up 抬头看，向上看

normal ['nɔːml] *adj.* 正常的，标准的   *e.g.* normal level 正常水平

breathing ['briːðɪŋ] *n.* 呼吸   *e.g.* abdominal breathing 腹式呼吸

come up 上来，起来

◆ Even if it is a long route, your perseverance will make it short.

reverse [rɪ'vɜːs] *v.* 互换（位置，功能），调换（位置）　***e.g.*** reverse roles 互换角色

repeat [rɪ'piːt] *v.* 重复（说、写或做）　***e.g.*** repeat after me 跟我读

on the other side 在另一边

same [seɪm] *adj.* 相同的　***e.g.*** same name 同名

length [leŋθ] *n.* 长度

the length of time 持续时间，时长

relieve [rɪ'liːv] *v.* 解除，减轻，缓和　***e.g.*** relieve pain 缓解疼痛

practise ['præktɪs] *v.* 练习（美式英语记作practice）　***e.g.*** practise yoga poses 练习瑜伽体式

against [ə'genst] *prep.* 倚靠，紧靠，碰　***e.g.*** lean against 靠在

top [tɒp] *adj.* （位置等）最高的，最上面的　***e.g.*** on the top floor 在顶楼

look down 向下看

at [æt] *prep.* 朝，向　***e.g.*** look at 看着，注视

in [ɪn] *prep.* 在……中　***e.g.*** in the past 在过去

final ['faɪnl] *adj.* 最终的　***e.g.*** final exam 期末考试

look ahead 向前看

make it easy 使其变得容易（或轻松）

◆即使是一条很长的路，你的毅力也会将它变短。

2.1.4　Vṛkṣāsana / Tree pose

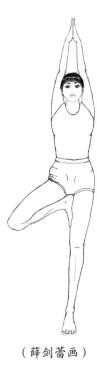

（薛剑蕾画）

Step-by-step Instructions

Begin in Mountain pose with your toes lifted and all four corners of your feet pressing into the earth.

Shift the weight of your body onto your left foot. Keep your left leg straight and steady.

Bend your right knee, catch hold of your right foot, and take the knee out to the right side.

◆ You don't cling to the object but just use it as a ladder to climb up. Once you have reached the roof you leave the ladder behind.

2.1.4 树式

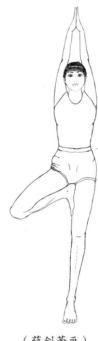

（薛剑蕾画）

步骤说明

以山式开始，脚趾抬起，每只脚上的四个角下压地面。

将身体重心转移到左脚上。保持左腿伸直、稳定。

屈右膝，抓握右脚，膝向右侧打开。

◆你不会抓住物体不放，而只是用它作为向上攀爬的梯子。一旦你爬上了屋顶，你就把梯子留在身后。

Bring the sole of your right foot to press against your left inner thigh with your heel near the groin. The sole of your right foot can also be placed below the knee on the inner lower leg if unable to place it above.

As you inhale, raise your arms out to the sides and overhead with the palms together or facing each other.

With your head straight, look straight ahead.

Hold this pose for 20 to 30 seconds.

Exhale, lower your right foot to the floor, take your arms down, and repeat on the other side.

Benefits

Tree pose can help

- · strengthen the thighs, calves, ankles and spine
- · improve coordination and brain functioning
- · improve sense of balance
- · improve blood circulation

Contraindications and Cautions

You should be careful with this pose if you have headache, insomnia or low blood pressure. Don't raise arms overhead if you have high blood pressure.

Words and Expressions / 词汇表达

tree [triː] *n.* 树   *e.g.* apple trees 苹果树

begin [bɪˈɡɪn] *v.* 开始   *e.g.* class begins 开始上课

shift [ʃɪft] *v.* 转移   *e.g.* shift away 把……移走

◆ To bring peace to the mind, watch and regulate the breath.

让右脚掌抵在左大腿内侧，脚跟靠近腹股沟。右脚掌如果不能置于膝盖以上，也可以放在膝盖以下小腿内侧。

随着吸气，手臂从两侧上举过头顶，合掌或掌心相对。

保持头部位置中正，直视前方。

在这个体式中保持20到30秒。

呼气，右脚落到地板上，手臂放下，换另一侧重复练习。

益处

树式能够帮助

- 强健大腿、小腿肚、脚踝和脊柱
- 提高协调能力，改善大脑功能
- 提升平衡感
- 促进血液循环

禁忌和注意事项

如果你有头痛、失眠或低血压，应当小心练习该体式。如果有高血压，手臂不要举过头顶。

weight [weɪt] *n.* （身体的）重心 *e.g.* shift your weight 转移你的重心
onto ['ɒntu] *prep.* 在……上，（身体重心）移向 *e.g.* fall onto 落在……上 shift...onto... 把……转移到……上

◆想让头脑平静，要观察和调节呼吸。

steady ['stedɪ] *adj.* 稳定的，稳固的   *e.g.* steady progress 稳步前进

catch hold of 抓住

take [teɪk] *v.* 引领   *e.g.* take...to... 把⋯⋯带到⋯⋯

press against 挤压，压在⋯⋯上

inner ['ɪnə] *adj.* 内部的   *e.g.* inner edge 内缘

near [nɪə] *prep.* 靠近，临近   *e.g.* near the yoga studio 靠近瑜伽馆

below [bɪ'ləʊ] *prep.* 在⋯⋯下面，低于   *e.g.* below normal 低于正常水平

unable [ʌn'eɪbəl] *adj.* 不能的   *e.g.* be unable to 无法，不能

place [pleɪs] *v.* 放置   *e.g.* place...on...把⋯⋯放在⋯⋯上

2.1.5   Vīrabhadrāsana I / Warrior pose I

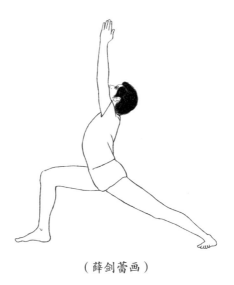

（薛剑蕾画）

◆ You can meditate on anything that will elevate you.

above [ə'bʌv] *prep.* 在……之上，高于　*e.g.* above normal 高于正常水平

raise [reɪz] *v.* 提起，抬起，举起　*e.g.* raise your head 抬起头

each other 彼此，互相

take...down（从高处）取下，拿下，放下

coordination [kəʊ,ɔ:dɪ'neɪʃn] *n.*（身体各部位的）协调能力　*e.g.* lack of coordination 缺乏协调能力

functioning ['fʌŋkʃənɪŋ] *n.* 运作，功能　*e.g.* social functioning 社会功能

sense of balance 平衡感

blood circulation 血液循环

2.1.5　战士一式

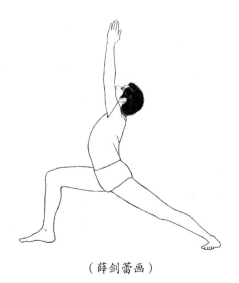

（薛剑蕾画）

◆你可以冥想于任何能提升你的东西。

Step-by-step Instructions

Start in Mountain pose. Walk or jump your feet about 1.2 metres (4 feet) apart.

Turn your right foot out 90 degrees. Turn your back foot slightly in and ground the outer edge, with the front heel aligned with the midline of the back foot.

Inhale, turn your pelvis, trunk and shoulders to the right. Square your hips and torso.

Exhale, bend your right knee directly over your right ankle to form a 90-degree angle so that your shin is perpendicular to the floor and your thigh is parallel to the floor.

Keep your back leg straight and firm. Make sure that the weight of your body does not fall on your right knee.

As you inhale, raise your arms out to the sides and overhead, with the palms together. As you exhale, draw your shoulders away from your ears.

Breathe evenly and stay in this pose for 20 to 30 seconds.

Inhale, straighten your legs to come up. Turn your trunk and both feet to face forward and then do on the other side.

Benefits

Warrior pose I can help

· relieve backache, lumbago and sciatica

· strengthen the shoulders, arms and back muscles

· strengthen and stretch the thighs, calves and ankles

◆ If you develop one idea through constant meditation, all other thoughts and desires will gradually die away.

步骤说明

由山式开始。双脚走或跳开约1.2米（4英尺）的距离。

左脚向外打开90度。后脚微微内收，脚外缘贴地，前脚脚跟与后脚中线处对齐。

吸气，骨盆、躯干及肩膀转动向右。髋部和躯干位置中正。

呼气，屈右膝到右脚踝正上方成90度角，这样，你的小腿胫骨垂直于地板，大腿与地板平行。

保持后腿蹬直、稳固。确保身体重心不落在右膝上。

随着吸气，手臂伸展向两侧并上举过头顶，合掌。随着呼气，双肩远离双耳。

均匀地呼吸，在这个体式中停留20到30秒。

吸气，双腿伸直起身。躯干和双脚转动面向前方，然后换另一侧练习。

益处

战士一式可以帮助

· 缓解背部疼痛、腰痛和坐骨神经痛

· 强健双肩、手臂及背部肌肉

· 强健并拉伸大腿、小腿肚和脚踝

◆如果你通过不断地冥想形成一个信念，所有其他的想法和欲望都会逐渐消失。

Contraindications and Cautions

This pose should be avoided if you have high blood pressure or heart disease.

Words and Expressions / 词汇表达

warrior ['wɒrɪə] *n.* 战士，勇士　*e.g.* a brave warrior 一位勇敢的武士

about [ə'baʊt] *adv.* 大约，将近　*e.g.* about 5 seconds 大约5秒

outer ['aʊtə] *adj.* 外部的　*e.g.* outer world 外在世界

front [frʌnt] *adj.* 前面的　*e.g.* front door 前门

align with 对齐，（尤指）使成一条直线

midline ['mɪdlaɪn] *n.* 中线，中间线　*e.g.* the midline of the lower abdomen 小腹中线

trunk [trʌŋk] *n.* （人体的）躯干　*e.g.* lift the trunk up 躯干上提

right [raɪt] *n.* 右边　*e.g.* to make a right 向右转弯

square [skweə] *v.* 挺直身子　*e.g.* square oneself 挺起胸膛

directly [də'rektli] *adv.* 直接地，正好地　*e.g.* directly above 正上方

◆ You need not fight to stop a habit. Just don't give it an opportunity to repeat itself.

禁忌和注意事项

如果有高血压或心脏病应避免练习该体式。

form [fɔ:m] *v.* 形成，构成　***e.g.*** form a right angle 形成一个直角

angle ['æŋgl] *n.* 角度　***e.g.*** a 30-degree angle 30度角

so that（引出结果）因此，所以

firm [fɜ:m] *adj.* 稳固的，强有力的　***e.g.*** a firm handshake 坚定有力的握手

fall on 落到，落在

stay [steɪ] *v.* 停留，保持　***e.g.*** stay at home 待在家里

forward ['fɔ:wəd] *adv.* 向前地（同forwards）　***e.g.*** bend forward 前屈

then [ðen] *adv.* 然后　***e.g.*** turn left first, then right 先左转后右转

do [du:] *v.* 做，干（某事）　***e.g.*** do homework 做家庭作业

avoid [ə'vɔɪd] *v.* 避免，避开　***e.g.*** avoid competition 规避竞争

◆你不需要拼命去改掉一个习惯。只要不给它重复的机会即可。

2.1.6 Garuḍāsana / Eagle pose

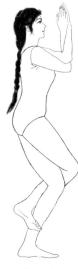

（薛剑蕾画）

Step-by-step Instructions

Stand in Mountain pose. Place your hands on your hips and bend your knees slightly.

Balancing on one foot, cross your right leg over your left and hook your right ankle behind your left calf.

Square your hips and torso. Elongate your spine and keep your tailbone in.

Inhale, bring your arms to chest level. Elbows bent and palms facing each other.

Exhale, cross the lower portion of your left upper arm on the right

---

◆ If you really want to go deep into meditation, take care to have a clean mind.

2.1.6 鹰式

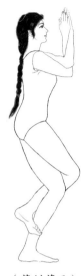

（薛剑蕾画）

步骤说明

山式站立。双手放于髋部，微屈膝。

将右腿交叉到左腿上，右脚踝勾住左小腿后方，保持平衡。

髋部和躯干位置中正。拉长脊柱，保持尾骨内收。

吸气，双臂抬至与胸部齐平。屈肘，掌心相对。

呼气，左大臂下端交叉于右二头肌。左小臂从右小臂前绕
过，合掌。右小臂要提供有力的支撑。

◆如果你真的想要深入冥想，注意保持头脑洁净。

bicep. Wrap your left forearm around the front of your right forearm and join the palms. The right forearm should offer firm support.

Inhale, raise your forearms perpendicular to the floor and raise them to eye level. Keep your eyes focused on a fixed point.

Hold this pose for 20 to 30 seconds, breathing evenly.

Release your arms and legs and return to Mountain pose. Relax with your eyes closed.

Then repeat the pose with the other leg on top, the other arm giving the support.

Benefits

Eagle pose can help

· strengthen the muscles and relax upper back

· loosen the joints of the shoulders, arms and legs

· improve concentration and sense of balance

Contraindications and Cautions

Do not do this pose if you have had a total hip replacement. Do it carefully or not at all if you have had knee injuries.

Words and Expressions / 词汇表达

eagle ['i:gl] *n.* 鹰 *e.g.* eagle eye 鹰眼，目光锐利的人

balance on 使（在某物上）保持平衡 *e.g.* balance on one leg 单腿平衡站立

cross [krɒs] *v.* 交叉，使相交 *e.g.* cross your arms 手臂交叉

◆ Even the so-called scientific discoveries and inventions are a result of concentration and meditation.

吸气，小臂保持垂直于地板向上抬，抬至视线高度。保持目光集中在一个固定的点上。

保持这个体式20到30秒，均匀地呼吸。

松开双臂和双腿，回到山式。双眼闭合，放松。

然后换另一条腿在上方，另一只手臂支撑，重复这个体式。

益处

鹰式能够帮助

·强健肌肉，放松上背部

·松解双肩、手臂和双腿的关节

·提升注意力和平衡感

禁忌和注意事项

如果你做了全髋关节置换手术，不要做这个体式。如有过膝关节损伤，做该体式时要小心或者干脆不做。

hook [hʊk] *v.* 钩住　 *e.g.* hook up 连接；勾搭

behind [bɪ'haɪnd] *prep.* 在……后面　 *e.g.* behind one's back 在某人背后

elongate ['i:lɒŋgeɪt] *v.* 拉长，使延长　 *e.g.* elongate the spine 拉长脊柱

◆甚至所谓的科学发现和发明都是专注和冥想的结果。

level ['levl] *n.* 水平，水平高度　*e.g.* energy level 能量水平

portion ['pɔːʃn] *n.* 部分　*e.g.* relevant portion 相关部分

upper ['ʌpə] *adj.* 上面的，上部的　*e.g.* upper back 上背部

wrap [ræp] *v.* 缠绕　*e.g.* wrap the bandage around the wound 用绷带包扎伤口

around [ə'raʊnd] *prep.* 围绕　*e.g.* around us 在我们周围

front [frʌnt] *n.* 前面，正面　*e.g.* in the front of 在……前面

join [dʒɔɪn] *v.* 连接，结合　*e.g.* join...to... 把……接到……上

offer ['ɒfə] *v.* 提供　*e.g.* offer something to somebody 为某人提供某物

support [sə'pɔːt] *n.* 支撑，支撑物　*e.g.* offer support to... 为……提供支撑

focus on 集中于，关注

fixed [fɪkst] *adj.* 固定的　*e.g.* fixed price 一口价

point [pɔɪnt] *n.* 点　*e.g.* focal point 焦点

◆ Tapas means "to burn or create heat." Anything burned out will be purified.

return to 回到

close [kləʊz] *v.* 关闭，闭合　*e.g.* close the door 关上门

the other 另一个，其他的

top [tɒp] *n.* 表面，上面　*e.g.* a desk top 桌面

give [gɪv] *v.*（与名词连用描述某一动作，意义与该名词相应的动词相同）　*e.g.* give a big smile 开心地笑

loosen ['luːsn] *v.* 使放松，使松弛　*e.g.* loosen up your muscles 放松肌肉

concentration [ˌkɒnsn'treɪʃn] *n.* 专心，专注　*e.g.* break one's concentration 打断某人的注意

total hip replacement 全髋关节置换手术

carefully ['keəfəlɪ] *adv.* 小心地，仔细地　*e.g.* drive carefully 小心驾驶

not at all 一点也不

◆Tapas的意思是"燃烧或产生热量"。任何燃烧掉的东西都会得到净化。

2.2 Sitting Poses

2.2.1 Daṇḍāsana / Staff pose

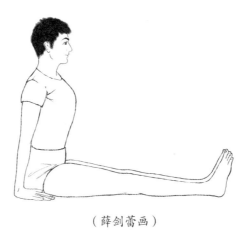

（薛剑蕾画）

Step-by-step Instructions

Begin in a seated position with your legs extended out in front.
Keep your thighs, knees, ankles and feet together.

Move the flesh of each buttock out to the side with your hands, so
that you are resting on the sitting bones.

Flex your feet and contract your front thigh muscles (quadriceps
muscles). Feel the hamstrings in the back of your legs stretch and
lengthen.

◆ We will actually be happy to receive pain if we keep in mind its purifying
effects.

2.2　坐立体式

2.2.1　手杖式

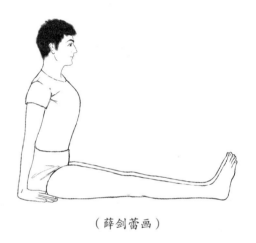

（薛剑蕾画）

步骤说明

由坐姿开始，双腿伸展向前。保持大腿、双膝、脚踝及双脚并拢。

双手将臀部两侧的肌肉向外拨开，帮助你坐在坐骨上。

勾脚并收紧大腿前侧肌肉（股四头肌）。感受腿后腘绳肌伸展及拉长。

◆如果我们牢记疼痛的净化作用，我们实际上会乐意接受疼痛。

Grounding your sitting bones, bring your torso to an upright position. You may sit on a folded blanket or bolster as needed to maintain your spine perpendicular to the earth.

Straighten your arms, bringing the shoulder blades back and down. Place your palms on the floor beside your hips, with your fingers pointing forward.

Your neck and head are straight. Look ahead at eye level.

Hold this pose for 20 to 30 seconds. Breathe evenly.

Feel the breath in your spine and notice how the spine elongates with each breath.

Benefits

Staff pose can help
 · tone the spinal and leg muscles
 · stretch the shoulders and chest
 · lengthen the ligaments of the legs and release the hamstrings

Contraindications and Cautions

Do not practise this pose if you have hamstring injury, ischial bursitis and lower back injury.

Words and Expressions / 词汇表达

staff [stɑːf] *n.* 拐杖，棍棒 *e.g.* a staff 一根拐杖

seated ['siːtɪd] *adj.* 就座的，坐下来的 *e.g.* seated posture 坐姿

position [pəˈzɪʃn] *n.* （坐、立的）姿态，姿势 *e.g.* a kneeling position 跪姿

◆ Although it is easy to bring pain to others, it is hard to accept it without striking back.

坐骨落地，躯干直立。你也可以根据需要坐在折叠的毯子或抱枕上以保持脊柱垂直于地面。

双臂伸直，肩胛骨向后并向下。手掌放在臀部两侧的地板上，手指指向前方。

头正颈直。水平目视前方。

保持这个体式20到30秒。均匀地呼吸。

感受气息在脊柱里流动，并觉察脊柱是如何随着每次呼吸拉长的。

益处

手杖式可以帮助

· 强健脊柱及腿部肌肉

· 拉伸双肩及胸腔

· 拉长腿部韧带，放松腘绳肌

禁忌和注意事项

如果腘绳肌受伤，有坐骨滑囊炎或下背部受伤，不要练习该体式。

---

move [mu:v] *v.* （使）改变位置，移动　*e.g.* move forward 向前移动
flesh [fleʃ] *n.* 肉，肉体　*e.g.* flesh and blood 血肉之躯
with [wɪð] *prep.* 用；使用　*e.g.* be filled with （被）用……充满

◆给别人带来痛苦很容易，但承受别人带来的痛苦不反击却很难。

sitting bone 坐骨 *e.g.* lift the sitting bones 抬起坐骨

flex [fleks] *v.* 屈伸（肌肉或身体的某部分） *e.g.* flex your fingers 活动手指

contract [kən'trækt] *v.* （使）收缩，缩小 *e.g.* contract your biceps 收紧肱二头肌

feel [fi:l] *v.* 感到 *e.g.* feel comfortable 感觉舒适

in the back of 在……的后面

lengthen ['leŋθən] *v.* 延长，拉长 *e.g.* lengthen your spine 拉长脊柱

upright ['ʌpraɪt] *adj.* 挺直的，直立的 *e.g.* an upright posture 直立的姿势

sit [sɪt] *v.* 坐 *e.g.* sit quietly 静静地坐着

folded [fəʊldɪd] *adj.* 折叠的 *e.g.* a folded chair 一把折叠的椅子

2.2.2　Jānu Śīrṣāsana / Head-to-knee pose

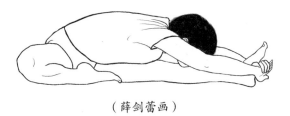

（薛剑蕾画）

Step-by-step Instructions

Sit in Staff pose. Bend your right knee out to the side and draw the heel back toward your perineum. Place the sole of your right foot against the left inner thigh and keep your right knee on the floor.

◆ Self-discipline is an aid to spiritual progress, whereas self-torture is an obstacle.

need [niːd] *v.* 需要　*e.g.* need to do something 需要做某事

maintain [meɪn'teɪn] *v.* 维持，保持　*e.g.* maintain health 保持健康

beside [bɪ'saɪd] *prep.* 在……旁边　*e.g.* beside the door 在门旁边

at eye level 在视线的水平高度

breath [breθ] *n.* 呼吸，气息，一口气　*e.g.* take a deep breath 深吸一口气

notice ['nəʊtɪs] *v.* 注意，觉察　*e.g.* I notice that...我觉察到……

spinal ['spaɪnl] *adj.* 脊柱的　*e.g.* spinal nerves 脊神经，脊髓神经

ligament ['lɪɡəmənt] *n.* 韧带　*e.g.* torn ligament 韧带撕裂

release [rɪ'liːs] *v.* 使不紧张，放松　*e.g.* release tension 释放紧张

injury ['ɪndʒəri] *n.* 损害，受伤　*e.g.* lung injury 肺损伤

2.2.2　单腿头碰膝式

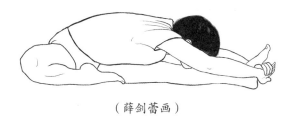

（薛剑蕾画）

步骤说明

手杖式坐立。屈右膝向外侧，将脚跟向后拉向会阴。右脚脚掌抵在左大腿内侧，保持右膝落在地板上。

◆自律是精神进步的助力，而自我折磨则是一种障碍。

Keep your left leg straight and point the toes of the left foot toward the ceiling.

On an inhalation, raise your arms overhead with the palms facing each other and lengthen your spine.

With an exhalation, slowly hinge forward from your hips and catch your left foot with both hands. Grip a yoga strap wrapped around your left foot if necessary.

Raise your head. Lift and open your chest.

Do not force yourself in the forward bend. Pause on inhalation and move on exhalation. Lengthen forward into a comfortable stretch.

Your lower belly should touch the left thigh before your chest and forehead rest on the left leg. Relax your shoulders, neck and head.

Your breath should remain smooth and relaxed as you hold this pose for 20 to 30 seconds.

To come out of the pose, inhale, lift your head and trunk up. Release your hands and come to Staff pose.

Repeat on the other side. Remain for the same length of time, then return to Staff pose.

Benefits

Head-to-knee pose can help
· stretch the hamstrings and the lumbosacral region of the spine
· stimulate the liver, the spleen and the kidneys
· reduce high blood pressure and relieve soreness and bloating in the breasts or abdomen
· relieve anxiety, fatigue, headache, menstrual discomfort and mild depression

---

◆ The mind should be purified first, then the senses can be controlled. Strict control over the senses alone will lead to difficulties instead of spiritual progress.

保持左腿伸直，左脚脚趾指向天花板。

随着吸气，手臂上举过头顶，掌心相对，拉长脊柱。

随着呼气，从髋部开始慢慢地向前折叠，双手抓住左脚。如有必要，将瑜伽伸展带缠绕在左脚并抓住。

抬头，上提并打开胸腔。

不要强迫自己前屈。吸气时停住，呼气时再动。身体向前拉伸进入舒展状态。

下腹部触碰到左大腿后，胸和额头依次贴放到左腿上。放松双肩、颈部和头部。

保持这个体式20到30秒，同时你的呼吸应当保持顺畅、放松。

退出体式时，吸气，抬头起身。双手解开，来到手杖式。

换另一侧重复练习。保持同样的时长，然后还原到手杖式。

益处

单腿头碰膝式能够帮助

· 拉伸腘绳肌及脊柱的腰骶区域

· 刺激肝脏、脾脏和肾脏

· 降低高血压并缓解乳房及腹部的疼痛和肿胀

· 缓解焦虑、疲劳、头痛、经期不适及轻度抑郁

◆首先要净化心灵，然后才能控制感官。只对感官严格控制会引向重重困难，而非精神进步。

Contraindications and Cautions

Do not practise this pose if you are clinically depressed or have diarrhea. Be careful with this pose if you have knee injury.

Words and Expressions / 词汇表达

perineum [ˌperɪˈniːəm] *n.* 会阴

on [ɒn] *prep.* 在……的时候　*e.g.* on an inhalation 随着一次吸气

inhalation [ˌɪnhəˈleɪʃn] *n.* 吸入，吸气　*e.g.* take a deep inhalation 深吸一口气

exhalation [ˌekshəˈleɪʃn] *n.* 吸入，吸气　*e.g.* a silent exhalation 无声的呼气

slowly [ˈsləʊli] *adv.* 缓慢地，慢慢地　*e.g.* walk slowly 慢慢地走

hinge [hɪndʒ] *v.* 给……装铰链　*e.g.* hinge on 取决于，以……为转移

from [frɒm] *prep.* 从，从……开始　*e.g.* start from scratch 从头开始

catch [kætʃ] *v.* 抓住，握住　*e.g.* catch hold of 抓住，紧握

grip [grɪp] *v.* 紧握，抓住　*e.g.* grip your arm 抓住你的手臂

necessary [ˈnesɪsəri] *adj.* 必要的，必需的　*e.g.* not necessary 不必要 if necessary 如果必要的话

open [ˈəʊpən] *v.* 打开　*e.g.* open the door 打开门

force oneself 强迫自己

forward bend 前屈

pause [pɔːz] *v.* 暂停，停顿　*e.g.* pause for breath 停下来喘口气

comfortable [ˈkʌmftəbl] *adj.* 舒适的，舒服的　*e.g.* comfortable clothes 舒适的衣服

◆ Speech should bring tranquility and be truthful, pleasant and beneficial.

禁忌和注意事项

如果你在临床上被诊断患有抑郁症，或腹泻，不要练习该体式。如果你的膝盖有伤，在练习该体式时要小心。

---

stretch [stretʃ] *n.*（四肢或身体的）舒展，伸展 *e.g.* have a good stretch 好好舒展一下身体

belly ['beli] *n.* 腹部 *e.g.* belly dance 肚皮舞

remain [rɪ'meɪn] *v.* 保持，停留 *e.g.* remain silent 保持沉默

smooth [smuːð] *adj.* 平稳的，连续而流畅的 *e.g.* smooth and steady 安稳的，平稳的

relaxed [rɪ'lækst] *adj.* 放松的，平静的 *e.g.* a relaxed atmosphere 轻松自在的氛围

come out of 从……中出来

come to 来到，到达

lumbosacral region ['lʌmbəu,seɪkrəl]['riːdʒən] 腰骶部

reduce [rɪ'djuːs] *v.* 减少，降低 *e.g.* reduce waste 减少浪费

soreness ['sɔːnəs] *n.* 疼痛，酸痛 *e.g.* waist soreness 腰酸

bloating ['bləʊtɪŋ] *n.*（身体）发肿；膨胀 *e.g.* abdominal bloating 腹胀

anxiety [æŋ'zaɪəti] *n.* 焦虑 *e.g.* relieve anxiety 缓解焦虑

fatigue [fə'tiːg] *n.* 疲劳，疲乏 *e.g.* visual fatigue 视觉疲劳

mild [maɪld] *adj.* 轻微的 *e.g.* mild fire 文火

clinically depressed 临床抑郁症的

◆言语应该带来平静，言语应当是诚实，令人愉快且有助益的。

2.2.3   Paśchimottānāsana / Seated Forward Bend pose

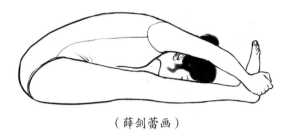

（薛剑蕾画）

Step-by-step Instructions

Sit in Staff pose. Make sure that you are sitting on your sitting bones and your weight is distributed equally on them. Put your palms on the floor beside your hips.

As you inhale, stretch your arms above your head, with the palms facing each other, and lengthen your torso upward. Relax your shoulders away from your ears.

As you exhale, draw your abdomen in, hinging forward from your hips with a long spine. Do not allow either buttock to rise off the floor.

With each inhalation, lengthen your spine; with each exhalation, release your torso forward.

Come as far forward as possible and then lower your arms to hold your calves, ankles or feet with both hands.

Renew the firm grounding of your sitting bones. Keep your torso lengthened and your head raised. Continue to experience the process of lengthening as you breathe in and descending as you breathe out.

◆ One should not speak what is true if it is not pleasant, nor what is pleasant if it is false.

2.2.3　坐立前屈式

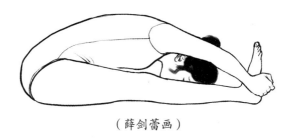

（薛剑蕾画）

步骤说明

手杖式坐立。确保坐在坐骨上，身体重量均匀分摊在上面。手掌放于臀部两侧的地板上。

随着吸气，手臂伸展过头顶，掌心相对，躯干拉长向上。双肩放松远离双耳。

随着呼气，腹部内收，保持脊柱拉长，从髋部开始向前折叠。不要让任何一侧臀部抬离地板。

随着每次吸气，拉长脊柱；随着每次呼气，放松躯干向前。

身体尽可能向前，然后手臂落下，双手抓住小腿肚、脚踝或双脚。

重新让坐骨稳定落地。保持躯干拉长，头部抬起。继续感受吸气时身体拉长，呼气时身体向下的过程。

◆一个人不应该说令人不悦的真话，也不应该说令人愉悦的假话。

In the final pose, your lower belly should touch the thighs first, and then your chest and forehead rest on your legs.

Remain in this pose for 20 seconds to start with and gradually increase the length of time you stay in the pose.

Benefits

Seated forward bend pose can help
· stretch the spine, shoulders and hamstrings
· increase flexibility in the hip joints
· stimulate and tone the entire abdominal and pelvic region
· calm the brain and relieve stress
· relieve the symptoms of menopause and menstrual discomfort

Contraindications and Cautions

People who suffer from herniated disc, sciatica or hernia should not practise this pose.

Words and Expressions / 词汇表达

distribute [dɪˈstrɪbjuːt] *v.* 使散开；使分布；分散　*e.g.* distribute evenly 均匀地分布

equally [ˈiːkwəli] *adv.* 相等地，同样　*e.g.* equally important 同等重要

put...on... 把……放在……上

allow...to... 允许……，让……

either [ˈiːðə] *adj.* （两者中）任一的　*e.g.* either way（两种情况中）

◆ Study does not just mean passing over the pages. It means trying to understand every word — studying with the heart.

在终极体式中，下腹部应当先贴放大腿，然后胸和额头依次贴腿。

一开始，在这个体式中保持20秒，然后逐渐延长在体式中停留的时间。

益处

坐立前屈式能够帮助

· 拉伸脊柱、肩膀及腘绳肌

· 提升髋关节的灵活度

· 刺激并强健整个腹盆区

· 平静大脑并缓解压力

· 缓解更年期症状及经期不适

禁忌和注意事项

患有椎间盘突出、坐骨神经痛或疝气的人不应该练习该体式。

不论发生哪种情况，无论怎样

rise [raɪz] *v.* 上升　*e.g.* rise from 从……升起

off [ɒf] *prep.* 离开　*e.g.* get off the bus 从公交车上下来，下车

as...as possible 尽量……，尽可能……

hold [həʊld] *v.* 拿着，抓住　*e.g.* hold hands 手拉手

renew [rɪ'njuː] *v.* 重新开始　*e.g.* renew the practice of meditation 重新

◆学习并不只是一页页翻书。它意味着努力去理解每一个词——用心学习。

开始练习冥想

continue [kən'tınjuː] *v.* 继续　　***e.g.*** continue working 继续工作

experience [ɪk'spɪərɪəns] *v.* 体验，感受　　***e.g.*** experience pain 感到痛苦

process ['prəʊses] *n.* 过程　　***e.g.*** learning process 学习过程

breathe in 吸入，吸气

descend [dɪ'send] *v.* 下降，下去，下来　　***e.g.*** descend step by step 逐步下降

breathe out 呼出，呼气

first [fɜːst] *adv.* 首先　　***e.g.*** rank first 名列第一

to start with 首先，作为开始

gradually ['grædʒuəli] *adv.* 逐步地，渐渐地　　***e.g.*** gradually decrease 逐渐减少

increase [ɪn'kriːs] *v.* 增加，提高　　***e.g.*** increase income 增加收入

◆ If you want to understand me fully, you must become me. Otherwise, you can understand me only according to your own capacity.

flexibility [ˌfleksə'bɪləti] *n.* 灵活性，弹性　　*e.g.* improve spinal flexibility 提高脊柱灵活性

entire [ɪn'taɪə] *adj.* 全部的，整个的　　*e.g.* entire life 一生

abdominal region 腹部区域，腹区

pelvic region 骨盆区

calm [kɑ:m] *v.* 使平静，使镇定　　*e.g.* calm down 平静下来

stress [stres] *n.* 压力，紧张　　*e.g.* mental stress 精神紧张，心理压力

symptom ['sɪmptəm] *n.* 症状　　*e.g.* clinical symptoms 临床症状

menopause ['menəpɔ:z] *n.* 更年期　　*e.g.* to reach the menopause 到更年期

suffer from 患……病，遭受

◆如果你想充分理解我，你必须成为我。否则，你只能根据自己的能力来理解我。

2.2.4   Gomukhāsana / Cow-face pose

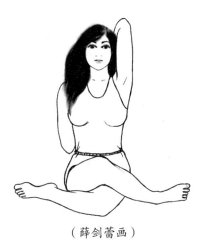

（薛剑蕾画）

Step-by-step Instructions

Sit in Staff pose. Bend your knees and rest your feet on the floor.

Draw your left leg under the right leg and bring the left heel to the outside of your right buttock.

Bring your right leg over the top of the left leg with the right heel close to the outside of your left buttock.

Press the tops of your feet into the earth as you squeeze your thighs together and line up the knees. You may sit on a folded blanket or a yoga block to keep your trunk upright and both sitting bones evenly grounded.

Raise your left arm, and bend it at the elbow. Your palm faces your back. Use your right hand to pull your left elbow closer to the midline of your head.

◆ Study is all right, but not for mere logic, quoting or fighting. Actually, it is only when you "quote" from your own experience that your words have weight.

2.2.4 牛面式

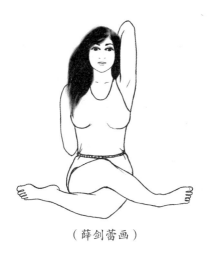

（薛剑蕾画）

步骤说明

手杖式坐立。屈膝，双脚落在地板上。

将左腿拉到右腿下面，把左脚跟带到右臀外侧。

将右腿放在左腿上方，右脚跟靠近左臀外侧。

大腿挤压在一起，双膝对齐，脚背压向地面。你可以坐在折叠的毯子或瑜伽砖上以保持躯干直立，两侧坐骨均匀落地。

左臂抬起向上，屈肘。掌心朝向后背。用右手拉动左肘，让左肘更贴近头部中线处。

◆学习是挺好的，但不只是为了逻辑、引用或争辩。实际上，只有当你"引用"自己的经验时，你的话才有分量。

Bend your right arm and bring it behind your back at the waist. The palm of the right hand faces away from your body. Centre your right hand between your shoulder blades.

Move both elbows backward bringing your hands close enough to grip the fingers of both hands. If you are not able to reach both hands, reach as far as you can with the help of a yoga strap.

Keep your head and neck straight.

Breathe deeply, relaxing into this pose for 20 seconds or longer.

To exit, release your arms and then uncross your legs. Now, repeat the pose by reversing your arms and legs.

Benefits

Cow-face pose can help

· improve posture

· alleviate tiredness, tension and anxiety

· relieve backache, sciatica, rheumatism and stiffness in the shoulders and neck

· stretch ankles, leg muscles, hips, thighs, shoulders and chest

Contraindications and Cautions

People who have trochanteric bursitis, serious shoulder or neck problems, or have had total hip or knee replacement should avoid this pose.

◆ Limit your reading and put into practice what you read.

屈右臂，来到背后腰部的位置。右手掌心背对身体。右手位于两侧肩胛骨中间。

双肘向后，双手足够靠近，让双手手指握紧在一起。如果双手触碰不到一起，可以借助瑜伽伸展带尽最大努力够触。

保持头正颈直。

深长地呼吸，放松进入到体式中保持20秒或更长。

退出时，松开双臂，然后解开双腿。现在，反转手臂和腿的位置，重复这个体式。

益处

牛面式能够帮助

·改善体态

·减轻疲劳、紧张和焦虑

·缓解背部疼痛、坐骨神经痛、风湿和肩颈僵硬

·拉伸脚踝、腿部肌肉、髋部、大腿、肩膀及胸部

禁忌和注意事项

患有大粗隆滑囊炎、存在严重的肩颈问题、曾做过全髋关节或膝关节置换术的人应避免该体式。

◆有限地阅读，将所读的付诸实践。

Words and Expressions / 词汇表达

cow [kaʊ] *n.* 奶牛，母牛

under ['ʌndə] *prep.* 在……下面 *e.g.* under your bed 在你的床下面

outside [ˌaʊt'saɪd] *n.* 外部，外侧 *e.g.* the outside of the house 房子的外部

close to 靠近，接近

squeeze [skwiːz] *v.* 挤，挤压 *e.g.* squeeze into 挤进

line up 对齐

at [æt] *prep.* 在（某处） *e.g.* at school 在学校

use...to... 使用……来……

pull [pʊl] *v.* 拉 *e.g.* pull the door open 拉开门

centre ['sentə] *v.* 把……放在中心处（美式英语记作center） *e.g.* centre around 以……为中心

backward ['bækwəd] *adv.* 向后地（同 backwards） *e.g.* fall backward 仰面摔倒

enough [ɪ'nʌf] *adv.* 足够地，充足地 *e.g.* good enough 足够好

2.2.5 Baddha Koṇāsana / Bound Angle pose

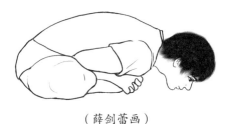

（薛剑蕾画）

◆ Even virtuous, meritorious deeds will bind you in some form or other if you do them with an egoistic feeling.

be able to 能够

reach [riːtʃ] *v.* 伸，伸手　*e.g.* reach out one's hand 伸出手

as far as you can 尽最大努力

with the help of 在……的帮助下

deeply ['diːpli] *adv.* 深深地　*e.g.* sigh deeply 长吁短叹

relax into 因放松下来而转入……

exit ['eksɪt] *v.* 出去，退出　*e.g.* exit from the classroom 离开教室

uncross [ʌn'krɒs] *v.* 使（原交叉的腿等）还原，使不交叉　*e.g.* uncross your arms 解开手臂

alleviate [ə'liːvɪeɪt] *v.* 减轻，缓和，缓解　*e.g.* alleviate back pain 缓解背部疼痛

tiredness ['taɪədnəs] *n.* 疲惫，疲倦　*e.g.* professional tiredness 职业倦怠

tension ['tenʃn] *n.* 紧张　*e.g.* nervous tension 神经紧张

serious ['sɪərɪəs] *adj.* 严重的　*e.g.* serious problems 严重的问题

2.2.5　束角式

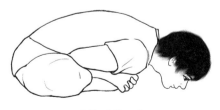

（薛剑蕾画）

◆如果你带着利己主义的心态行事，即使是行善立功，也会以某种形式束缚你。

Step-by-step Instructions

Sit in Staff pose. Bend your legs one at a time, taking your knees out and your heels toward the perineum. Press the soles of your feet together.

If your knees are higher than your hips or your back is rounded, sit up on a folded blanket or bolster.

Hold your big toes with your thumbs, index and middle fingers, or interlock your fingers and clasp around the feet.

As you inhale, lengthen your spine, draw your shoulders back and lift your ribcage up.

As you exhale, allow your lengthened torso to gradually bend forward from the hinge of your hips.

Grounding your sitting bones, descend as far as possible with a neutral spine.

You can also rest your hands or forearms onto the earth, shoulder-width apart, allowing your awareness to turn inward.

Stay in this pose for 20 to 30 seconds, breathing evenly. Remaining in the pose for an extended length of time will slowly release tightness in the hips.

Release your hands and stretch your legs out to Staff pose.

Benefits

Bound Angle pose can help
  · tone the spine, abdominal organs and pelvic organs
  · stimulate the heart and improve blood circulation
  · reduce menstrual discomfort and irregular periods

◆ Only the light of understanding will remove the darkness of ignorance.

步骤说明

手杖式坐立。依次屈腿，双膝向外展开，脚跟朝向会阴。双脚脚掌压在一起。

如果双膝高于髋部或背部拱起，端坐在折叠的毯子或抱枕上。

用大拇指、食指和中指抓住大脚趾，或者十指交叉扣紧双脚。

随着吸气，拉长脊柱，双肩向后，胸腔上提。

随着呼气，让拉长的躯干以髋部为折点，逐渐地向前折叠。

坐骨落地，保持脊柱中正，身体尽量向下沉。

你也可以让双手或小臂停留在地面上，打开与肩同宽，让你的觉知转向内部。

在这个体式中保持20到30秒，均匀地呼吸。在该体式中保持更长的时间会慢慢地释放掉髋部的紧绷感。

双手松开，双腿伸出去，回到手杖式。

益处

束角式能够帮助

· 强健脊柱、腹部及盆腔器官

· 刺激心脏，改善血液循环

· 减少经期不适及月经不规律

◆只有理解之光才能驱除无明的黑暗。

· stretch the inner thighs, groin and knees

· alleviate urinary system disorder

· prevent sciatica and hernia

· relieve mild depression, anxiety, fatigue and symptoms of menopause

Contraindications and Cautions

Perform Bound Angle pose with blankets under the outer thighs if you have groin or knee injury. Sit against a wall if you have asthma, bronchitis or heart disease.

Words and Expressions / 词汇表达

bound [baʊnd] *adj.* 受约束的，被限制的 *e.g.* be bound by 受……约束

one at a time 一次一个

high [haɪ] *adj.* 高的 *e.g.* a high mountain 一座高山

than [ðæn] *prep.* （用以引出比较的第二部分）比 *e.g.* smaller than... 比……小

round [raʊnd] *v.* 使变圆 *e.g.* round off 圆满结束；圆满完成

sit up 端坐，坐直身子

interlock [ˌɪntəˈlɒk] *v.* 互锁，扣紧 *e.g.* interlock your fingers 十指交叉

clasp [klɑːsp] *v.* 紧抱，扣紧 *e.g.* clasp hands 紧握双手

hinge [hɪndʒ] *n.* 枢纽，转折点 *e.g.* the hinge of history 历史的转折点

◆ Yoga is neither for a person who has gained the light nor for a totally ignorant person who doesn't bother to know anything. It is for a person in between. It is to dispel this ignorance that yoga is practiced.

·拉伸大腿内侧、腹股沟及双膝

·缓解泌尿系统紊乱

·预防坐骨神经痛和疝气

·缓解轻度抑郁、焦虑、疲劳及更年期症状

禁忌和注意事项

如果你的腹股沟或膝盖有伤，做束角式时可以在大腿外侧下方垫毯子。如果你有哮喘、支气管炎或心脏病，靠墙坐立。

as far as possible 尽量，尽可能

neutral ['njuːtrəl] *adj.* 中和的，不引起变化的　*e.g.* neutral budget 中性预算

awareness [ə'weənəs] *n.* 意识，觉知　*e.g.* environmental awareness 环境意识

inward ['ɪnwəd] *adv.* 向内地（同inwards）　*e.g.* push inward 向内推

tightness ['taɪtnəs] *n.* 紧绷，不适　*e.g.* chest tightness 胸闷

prevent [prɪ'vent] *v.* 预防，防止　*e.g.* prevent cancer 预防癌症

perform [pə'fɔːm] *v.* 做　*e.g.* perform miracles 创造奇迹

◆瑜伽既不是为业已证悟的人准备的，也不是为懒于学习的全然无明之辈所准备。它是为处在中间的人准备的。习练瑜伽就是为了消除无明。

2.2.6 Upaviṣṭha Koṇāsana / Seated Angle pose

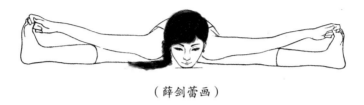

（薛剑蕾画）

Step-by-step Instructions

Sit in Staff pose. Separate your legs and stretch them out toward your heels.

Place your hands beside your hips. Press your palms down on the floor to raise your pelvis up off the floor and slide it forward to widen the distance between your legs.

Rotate your thighs to the front so that the kneecaps and toes face the ceiling. Keep your legs extended and press your thighs and shinbones into the floor.

Lift your spine and chest, moving your shoulder blades in.

Catch your big toes with respective thumbs and index and middle fingers.

Inhale, lengthen your spine; exhale, bend forward. Increase the forward bend on each exhalation until you feel a comfortable stretch in the backs of your legs.

In the final pose, you can extend your torso and rest your abdomen, chest and chin on the floor.

Keep both sitting bones evenly grounded and stay in this pose for

◆ The ego is the reflection of the true self on the mind. The self will always be falsely represented by the ego until our ignorance is removed.

2.2.6　坐角式

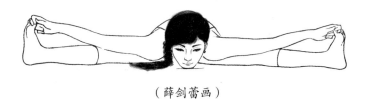

（薛剑蕾画）

步骤说明

手杖式坐立。双腿分开，向脚跟方向伸展。

双手放在臀部两侧。手掌下压地板，以此让骨盆抬离地板并向前滑动增大双腿之间的距离。

将大腿转动向前，使髌骨和脚趾朝向天花板。保持双腿伸展，大腿和胫骨下压地板。

脊柱和胸部上提，肩胛骨内收。

分别用大拇指、食指和中指抓握大脚趾。

吸气，拉长脊柱；呼气，身体前屈。随着每次呼气，增加前屈的深度，直到你感到双腿后侧得到舒适的拉伸。

在终极体式中，你可以让躯干伸展，腹部、胸部及下巴停留在地板上。

保持两侧坐骨均匀落地，在这个体式中停留20到30秒，正常呼吸。

◆自我是真我在头脑中的反映。在无明被消除之前，真我将一直被自我错误地代表。

20 to 30 seconds with normal breathing.

Inhale, raise your trunk off the floor and release the hold on your feet. Slowly slide your legs back to Staff pose and relax.

Benefits

Seated Angle pose can help
- stretch the hamstrings and relieve sciatica
- stimulate the ovaries and regularize the menstrual flow
- improve the blood circulation in the pelvic region
- strengthen the spine and massage the abdominal organs

Contraindications and Cautions

Sit up high on a folded blanket and keep your torso relatively upright in case of lower-back injury.

Words and Expressions / 词汇表达

separate ['sepəreɪt] v. 使（分离），分开 e.g. separate A from B 将A和B分离开

raise up 举起，抬起

slide [slaɪd] v. 滑动 e.g. slide down 滑下，往下滑

distance ['dɪstəns] n. 距离，间隔 e.g. at a distance 离一段距离

rotate [rəʊ'teɪt] v. 使旋转，使转动 e.g. rotate around 围绕……旋转

respective [rɪ'spektɪv] adj. 分别的 e.g. their respective characteristics 它们各自的特色

◆ I often refer to these two "I"s as the little "i" and the capital "I". What is the difference? Just a small dot, a little blemish of ego.

吸气，躯干抬离地板，松开对双脚的抓握。双腿慢慢滑动回到手杖式，放松。

益处

坐角式能够帮助

· 拉伸腘绳肌并缓解坐骨神经痛

· 促进卵巢功能并调节月经

· 促进骨盆区域的血液循环

· 强健脊柱，按摩腹部器官

禁忌和注意事项

以防下背部受伤，高坐在折叠的毯子上，保持躯干相对直立。

---

hold [həʊld] *n.* 抓，握 *e.g.* take hold of 抓住，握着

regularize ['reɡjələraɪz] *v.* 调整，调节 *e.g.* regularize heart beat 调节心跳

menstrual flow 月经

massage ['mæsɑːʒ] *v.* 按摩 *e.g.* massage aching muscles 按摩疼痛的肌肉

relatively ['relətɪvlɪ] *adv.* 相对地 *e.g.* relatively safe 相对安全

in case of 如果发生

◆我常把这两个"I"（我）称为小写的i和大写的I。有什么区别呢？区别只是一个小点，一点自我的瑕疵。

2.3   Prone Poses

2.3.1   Makarāsana / Crocodile pose[5]

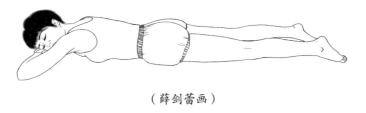

（薛剑蕾画）

Step-by-step Instructions

Begin lying on your abdomen with your right hand on top of your left hand.

Rest your right cheek on the back of your hands with your gaze directed toward your left elbow.

Extend your legs with your feet hip-width apart and the tops of your feet on the floor.

Let your legs and arms relax completely and release the weight of your body onto the floor.

Soften your abdomen; allow it to expand against the floor as you inhale and to contract as you exhale.

Close your eyes and sense the contact of your body with the floor.

Remain in this position for several breaths.

◆ The capital "I" is just one pure stroke, just as the highest truth is always simple and pure. What limits us and makes us little? Just the dot. All the practice of yoga are just to remove that dot.

2.3　俯卧体式

2.3.1　鳄鱼式⑤

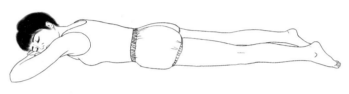

（薛剑蕾画）

步骤说明

以俯卧开始，右手叠放于左手上。

右脸颊贴放在手背上，目光看向左肘。

双腿伸展，双脚打开与髋同宽，脚背贴地。

让双腿和双臂完全放松，身体的重量释放到地板上。

腹部柔软下来；让它随着吸气时扩张触碰地板，呼气时收缩。

闭上双眼，感受身体与地板的接触。

在这个姿势中保持几个呼吸。

　　◆大写的"I"（我）只是纯净的一笔，正如至高的真理永远是简单而纯粹的。是什么限制了我们，令我们渺小？只是一个点。所有的瑜伽练习都是为了去掉那个点。

Now, repeat the pose by switching the position of your hands with your left hand on top, resting your left cheek on the back of your hands and gazing at your right elbow.

Benefits

Crocodile pose can help
· relax your whole body and mind
· free the body from tension and soothe the nerves

Contraindications and Cautions

Women during pregnancy should avoid this pose.

Words and Expressions / 词汇表达

crocodile ['krɒkədaɪl] *n.* 鳄鱼

lie [laɪ] *v.* 躺，平躺　*e.g.* lie on your side 侧卧

on [ɒn] *prep.* 由……支撑着　*e.g.* lie on your back 仰卧　lie on one's abdomen/stomach 俯卧　on top of 在……之上

direct [daɪ'rekt] *v.* 指向　*e.g.* direct...at...把……对准（某方向或某人）

let [let] *v.* 允许，让　*e.g.* Let me help you. 让我来帮你吧。

completely [kəm'pliːtli] *adv.* 完全地，全然地　*e.g.* completely different 完全不同

soften ['sɒfn] *v.* 使变柔软　*e.g.* soften up 使软化

expand [ɪk'spænd] *v.* 扩张，膨胀　*e.g.* expand your chest 扩展胸腔

sense [sens] *v.* 感觉，感到　*e.g.* sense danger 感觉到危险

contact ['kɑːntækt] *n.* 接触　*e.g.* eye contact 目光接触

◆ We attach ourselves to pleasure because we expect happiness from it, forgetting that happiness is always in us as the true self.

现在，交换双手位置让左手在上，左脸颊贴放在手背上，看向右肘，重复该体式。

益处

鳄鱼式能够帮助

· 放松你的整个身心

· 让身体摆脱紧张并舒缓神经

禁忌和注意事项

孕期女性应避免该体式。

---

several ['sevrəl] *adj.* 几个的　*e.g.* several days 好几天

switch [swɪtʃ] *v.* 对调，改变（方向等）　*e.g.* switch roles 互换角色

gaze at 盯住，凝视

whole [həʊl] *adj.* 整个的，全部的　*e.g.* whole body 全身

mind [maɪnd] *n.* 头脑，心思　*e.g.* on one's mind 挂在心上，惦念

free...from... 使免于……，使摆脱……

soothe [suːð] *v.* 缓和，缓解　*e.g.* soothe...away 消除，解除

nerve [nɜːv] *n.* 神经（nerves：神经，神经紧张）　*e.g.* calm one's nerves 平静情绪

woman ['wʊmən] *n.* 妇女，女性　*e.g.* a Chinese woman 一个中国女人

pregnancy ['pregnənsi] *n.* 怀孕，孕期　*e.g.* during pregnancy 在怀孕期间

◆我们寻欢作乐，因为我们期望从中获得快乐，却忘了快乐作为真正的自我一直在我们心中。

2.3.2 Aṣṭāṅga Namaskāra / Eight-limbed Salutation pose

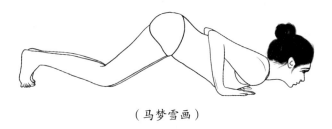

（马梦雪画）

Step-by-step Instructions

Start in Downward-facing Dog pose (see page 165). Keep your hands and feet in place.

Lower your knees to the floor while lifting your pelvis upward. Place your chest and chin on the floor with your hands beneath the shoulders.

Eight points of your body touch the ground: toes of both feet, two knees, chest, two hands and chin.

Keep your buttocks, hips and abdomen elevated. Tighten the muscles at your navel centre.

The breath is held out in this pose. There is no respiration.

Inhale, move on to the next pose.

Benefits

Eight-limbed Salutation pose can help

· strengthen the leg and arm muscles

· stretch the chest

· exercise the region of the spine between the shoulder blades

---

◆ No one can ever give us happiness or unhappiness. One can only reflect or distort our own inner happiness.

2.3.2　八体投地式

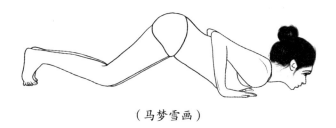

（马梦雪画）

步骤说明

以下犬式（见本书第165页）开始。双手和双脚固定不动。

保持骨盆上提的同时双膝落向地板。胸和下巴点地，双手在肩膀下方。

身体八个点触地：双脚脚趾，双膝，胸部，双手和下巴。

保持臀部、髋部和腹部抬高。收紧肚脐中心的肌肉。

在这个体式中外屏息（即呼气后屏息）。不进行呼吸。

吸气，进入到下一个体式。

益处

八体投地式能够帮助

・强健腿部和手臂的肌肉

・伸展胸腔

・锻炼肩胛骨之间的脊柱区域

◆没有人能给我们快乐或不悦，只能反映或扭曲我们自己内心的快乐。

Contraindications and Cautions

Do not practise this pose if you have high blood pressure, heart conditions or serious back problems.

Words and Expressions / 词汇表达

salutation [ˌsæljuˈteɪʃn] *n.* 致意，致意的动作　*e.g.* Sun Salutation 拜日式

downward [ˈdaʊnwəd] *adv.* 向下地（同downwards）　*e.g.* point downward 向下指

dog [dɒg] *n.* 狗

keep...in place 固定住，保持

beneath [bɪˈniːθ] *prep.* 在……之下　*e.g.* the ground beneath your feet 你脚下的土地

2.3.3　Bhujaṅgāsana / Cobra pose

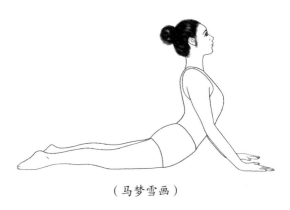

（马梦雪画）

◆ Every action will leave its result; every cause will bear its effect.

禁忌和注意事项

如果你有高血压、心脏病或严重的背部问题，不要练习该体式。

---

elevated ['elɪveɪtɪd] *adj.* 抬高的　*e.g.* elevated railway 高架铁路

tighten ['taɪtn] *v.* 收紧，使变紧　*e.g.* tighten the yoga strap 拉紧瑜伽伸展带

there is... 有（表示存在）

respiration [ˌrespə'reɪʃn] *n.* 呼吸　*e.g.* artificial respiration 人工呼吸

move on to 开始做（别的事），移到

next [nekst] *adj.* 紧接在后的，下一个　*e.g.* next week 下周

exercise ['eksəsaɪz] *v.* 锻炼，练习　*e.g.* exercise regularly 定期锻炼

2.3.3　眼镜蛇式

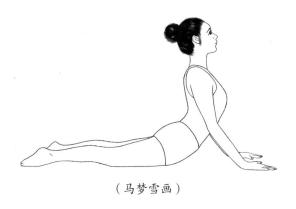

（马梦雪画）

◆行动即有果；有因必有果。

Step-by-step Instructions

Lie flat on your stomach with your legs straight and feet together (or hip-width apart). Extend your arms overhead with your forehead resting on the earth.

Position your palms directly under your shoulders with your fingers spread wide apart and the middle fingers pointing forward. Your upper arms stay in contact with the sides of your ribcage.

As you inhale, grounding your pelvis, legs and feet, slowly raise your head and neck, push your hands into the floor and lift your back off the ground vertebra by vertebra.

Roll your shoulders back and down. Straighten your arms or slightly bend your elbows, depending on the flexibility of your back.

Raise your head up and look up.

Breathe normally through your nose. Remain in this pose for 20 to 30 seconds.

As you exhale, release down by bending your elbows and lowering your abdomen, chest, and forehead to the floor. Rest for several breaths, relaxing all the muscles of the back of your body.

Benefits

Cobra pose can help
- improve and deepen breathing
- keep the spine supple and healthy, and remove backache
- tone the ovaries and uterus, and relieve menstrual disorders
- stimulate abdominal organs and alleviate constipation

◆ Life is experienced by the mind through the body. The body is only a vehicle or instrument.

步骤说明

俯卧下来，双腿伸直，双脚并拢（或打开与髋同宽）。手臂伸展过头顶，额头停留在地面上。

手掌置于肩膀正下方，手指大大地分开，中指指向前方。大臂贴胸腔两侧。

随着吸气，保持骨盆、双腿及双脚贴地，慢慢抬起头部和颈部，双手推地，让后背脊椎一节一节地抬离地面。

双肩向后并向下转动。根据背部的灵活度伸直手臂或微屈手肘。

抬头向上看。

通过鼻子正常呼吸。在这个体式中保持20到30秒。

随着呼气，通过屈肘，腹部、胸部和前额落地，让身体放松向下。休息几个呼吸，放松身体背部所有肌肉。

益处

眼镜蛇式能够帮助

· 改善和加深呼吸

· 保持脊柱灵活健康并消除背部疼痛

· 调理卵巢和子宫，缓解月经紊乱

· 刺激腹部器官，缓解便秘

◆心灵通过身体体验生活。身体只是一种媒介或工具。

Contraindications and Cautions

Women should not practise this pose during pregnancy. People with peptic ulcer, hernia or intestinal tuberculosis can only practise this pose under the supervision of a competent teacher.

Words and Expressions / 词汇表达

cobra ['kəʊbrə] *n.* 眼镜蛇　*e.g.* king cobra 眼镜王蛇

flat [flæt] *adv.*（尤指贴着另一表面）平直地　*e.g.* lie flat 平躺

position [pə'zɪʃn] *v.* 安置, 把……放在适当位置　*e.g.* position the vase with care 小心放置花瓶

wide [waɪd] *adv.* 充分地　*e.g.* wide open 完全打开的

in contact with 与……接触

roll [rəʊl] *v.* 转动　*e.g.* roll your eyes 转动眼珠

depend on 取决于

through [θruː] *prep.* 通过, 经由　*e.g.* breathe through your nostrils 通过鼻孔呼吸

禁忌和注意事项

女性在孕期不应练习该体式。患有消化性溃疡、疝气或肠结核的人只有在有能力的老师的监督指导下才能练习这个体式。

rest [rest] *v.* 休息　　***e.g.*** rest for a moment 休息片刻

back [bæk] *n.* 后部，背面　　***e.g.*** the back of... ……的背面

deepen ['diːpən] *v.* （使）变深，加深　　***e.g.*** deepen the understanding of 深化理解

supple ['sʌpl] *adj.* 灵活的，柔软的　　***e.g.*** supple knees 灵活的双膝

healthy ['helθi] *adj.* 健康的　　***e.g.*** a healthy diet 健康饮食

only ['əʊnlɪ] *adv.* 只有，仅仅　　***e.g.*** only when 只有当……的时候才能

under the supervision of 在……的监督下

competent ['kɒmpɪtənt] *adj.* 有能力的，能胜任的　　***e.g.*** a competent teacher 一位称职的老师

2.3.4 Śalabhāsana / Locust pose[6]

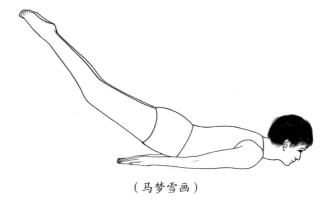

（马梦雪画）

Step-by-step Instructions

Lying prone with your chin on the floor and your legs and feet together.

Tuck your arms underneath your body, elbows close together and palms facing the floor or in gentle fists.

Take a slow and deep breath and withhold the breath inside, contract the muscles of your lower extremities and lift both legs up to a comfortable height.

Lengthen your lower back while extending out the legs through the feet. Keep your knees straight.

Remain in this pose for as long as you can retain the breath.

On the next exhalation, bring your legs down slowly, release your hands, and relax the muscles of your whole body.

◆ You are your own best friend as well as your worst enemy.

2.3.4 蝗虫式^⑥

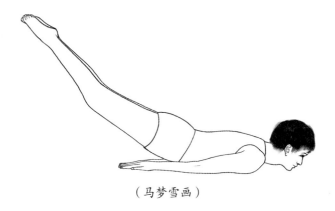

（马梦雪画）

步骤说明

俯卧，下巴点地，双腿双脚并拢。

手臂收拢到身体下面，手肘紧靠在一起，掌心朝向地板或轻柔握拳。

深长缓慢地吸一口气，屏住呼吸，收紧下肢肌肉，双腿抬起到舒适的高度。

通过双脚伸展双腿的同时拉长下背部。保持双膝伸直。

呼吸能保持多久，在体式中就停留多久。

下一次呼气时，慢慢放下双腿，松开双手并放松全身肌肉。

◆你是自己最好的朋友，也是自己最大的敌人。

Benefits

Locust pose can help
- · strengthen the lower back, arms and abdominal muscles
- · tone the viscera, remove indigestion, and relieve constipation
- · relieve backache, mild sciatica and slipped disc
- · tone the sympathetic nervous system
- · promote elasticity of the lungs

Contraindications and Cautions

This pose should be avoided by people with a weak heart, high blood pressure, hernia or gastrointestinal ulcer. Women should not practise this pose during menstruation and pregnancy. Those that have lower back problems should begin with lifting legs one at a time to a comfortable height.

Words and Expressions / 词汇表达

locust ['ləʊkəst] *n.* 蝗虫 *e.g.* a swarm of locusts 一群蝗虫

prone [prəʊn] *adj.* 俯卧的 *e.g.* prone position 卧姿

underneath [ˌʌndəˈniːθ] *prep.* 在……底下 *e.g.* underneath the table 在桌子底下

gentle ['dʒentl] *adj.* 温和的，轻柔的 *e.g.* a gentle breeze 微风

fist [fɪst] *n.* 拳头 *e.g.* make a fist 握拳

take [teɪk] *v.*（与名词连用，表示举动、动作等） *e.g.* take a look 看一眼

◆ All our so-called pleasures bring in the fear of losing them.

益处

蝗虫式能够帮助

- 强健下背部、手臂和腹部肌肉
- 调理脏腑，消除消化不良，缓解便秘
- 缓解背部疼痛、轻度坐骨神经痛和椎间盘突出
- 调节交感神经系统
- 提升肺部弹性

禁忌和注意事项

有心脏衰弱、高血压、疝气或消化道溃疡的人应避免这个体式。女性在经期和孕期不应练习这个体式。下背部有问题的人开始时应当单次只抬一条腿到舒适的高度。

---

slow [sləʊ] *adj.* 慢的　***e.g.*** slow speed 慢速，低速

deep [diːp] *adj.* 深的　***e.g.*** deep water 深水

withhold [wɪð'həʊld] *v.* 保留，抑制（情感或反应等）　***e.g.*** withhold from 忍住不做

inside [ˌɪn'saɪd] *adv.* 在里面　***e.g.*** go inside 进去

lower extremities 下肢

as long as 只要，和……一样长

retain [rɪ'teɪn] *v.* 保持　***e.g.*** retain respect 保留尊严

◆ 所有我们所谓的快乐都会带来失去它们的恐惧。

viscera ['vɪsərə] *n.* 内脏，脏腑　*e.g.* abdominal viscera 腹部脏器

sympathetic nervous system 交感神经系统

promote [prə'məʊt] *v.* 提升，促进　*e.g.* promote economic growth 促
进经济增长

2.3.5　Dhanurāsana / Bow pose

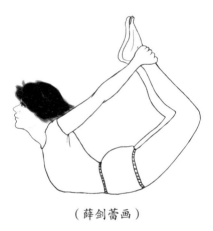

（薛剑蕾画）

Step-by-step Instructions

From the prone position, bring your chin to the floor and place
your arms along the sides of your body with your palms up and feet
hip-width apart.

Bend your knees, and bring your heels toward your buttocks.
Reach back to hold your ankles from the outside.

Inhale, press the feet back into your hands, feel the traction in your

---

◆ Real pleasure comes from detaching ourselves completely from the entire
world, in standing aloof—making use of the world as a master of it.

elasticity [ˌiːlæ'stɪsəti] *n. 弹性，灵活性*　***e.g.*** high elasticity *高弹性*
menstruation [ˌmenstru'eɪʃn] *n. 月经*

2.3.5　弓式

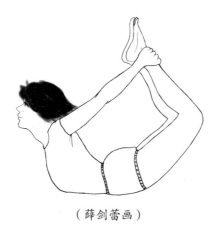

（薛剑蕾画）

步骤说明

由俯卧开始，下巴触地，手臂放于身体两侧，掌心向上，双脚打开与髋同宽。

屈膝，并将脚跟带向臀部。双手向后从外侧抓握脚踝。

吸气，双脚向后压入手中，感受手臂和双肩的牵引，同时将上半身和下半身向上提拉。

◆真正的快乐来自完全超脱整个世界，置身其外——作为主宰者利用世界。

arms and shoulders, and lift your upper and lower body simultaneously.

Keep a firm grip on your ankles and use a resistance between the legs and the arms to help raise your legs and chest further.

Try to keep your legs and feet parallel to each other, imagining your thighs are pressing inward against a yoga block.

Rest your lower abdomen on the floor. Lift your head and look up.

Breathe and relax with the breath.

Remain in this pose as long as you can comfortably do so.

To come out of the pose, lower your knees and chest first. Then bring your hands and legs down and stretch flat on the ground.

Benefits

Bow pose can help

· massage the liver, abdominal organs and muscles

· reduce excess fat around the abdominal area

· improve the digestive, excretory and reproductive systems

· control diabetes and alleviate menstrual disorders

· extend the spine and remove stiffness

· correct hunching of the upper back

· strengthen leg muscles, especially the thighs

Contraindications and Cautions

Don't practise Bow pose if you have high blood pressure, a weak heart, hernia, colitis, peptic or duodenal ulcers. Avoid the practice of this pose before bed as it can stimulate the adrenal glands and the sympathetic nervous system.

◆ When someone can't adapt himself to his known family, how can he be expected to adapt to an unknown group? A known devil is much better than an unknown one.

紧紧抓握脚踝，使用双腿与手臂之间的抗力帮助双腿及胸腔向上提得更高。

尽量保持双腿和双脚互相平行，想象大腿向内压一块瑜伽砖。

下腹部停留在地板上。抬头向上看。

呼吸，跟随呼吸放松。

在舒适的前提下保持该体式。

退出体式时，双膝和胸部先落下。然后，双手和双腿落下，身体平直伸展。

益处

弓式能够帮助

· 按摩肝脏、腹部器官和肌肉

· 减少腹部周围多余的脂肪

· 改善消化、排泄和生殖系统

· 控制糖尿病并缓解经期紊乱

· 延展脊柱，消除僵硬感

· 矫正上背部驼背

· 强健腿部肌肉，尤其是大腿

禁忌和注意事项

如果你有高血压、心脏衰弱、疝气、结肠炎、消化性溃疡或十二指肠溃疡，不要练习弓式。睡前不要做这个动作，因为它会刺激肾上腺和交感神经系统。

◆当一个人不能适应他所熟悉的家庭时，怎能期望他适应一个不熟悉的群体呢？熟悉的魔鬼比不熟悉的要好得多。

Words and Expressions / 词汇表达

bow [bəʊ] *n.* 弓   *e.g.* bow and arrow 弓箭

traction ['trækʃn] *n.* 牵引，拉力   *e.g.* traction force 牵引力

simultaneously [ˌsɪml'teɪnɪəsli] *adv.* 同时地   *e.g.* improve simultaneously 同步提高

grip [ɡrɪp] *n.* 紧握，抓住   *e.g.* get a grip on 抓住，把握关键

resistance [rɪ'zɪstəns] *n.* 阻力，抗力   *e.g.* water resistance 水阻力

between...and... ……和……之间

further ['fɜːðə] *adv.* 进一步地，更远地   *e.g.* to further explain 进一步解释

comfortably ['kʌmftəbli] *adv.* 舒服地，舒适地   *e.g.* sit comfortably 舒服地坐着

excess [ɪk'ses] *adj.* 过量的，过剩的   *e.g.* excess baggage 超额行李

2.3.6   Maṇḍūkāsana / Frog pose

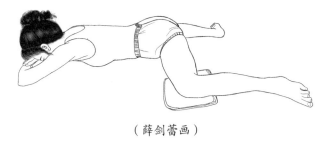

（薛剑蕾画）

◆ Wherever we are, we have to learn to handle things properly.

fat [fæt] *n.* 脂肪，肥肉　*e.g.* low fat 低脂

area ['eərɪə] *n.* 区域，部位　*e.g.* chest area 胸部

excretory system 排泄系统

control [kən'trəʊl] *v.* 控制，管理　*e.g.* control oneself 控制自己

correct [kə'rekt] *v.* 纠正，修正　*e.g.* correct mistakes 纠正错误

hunch [hʌntʃ] *v.* 耸肩，弓背　*e.g.* hunch over the desk 伏在桌上

especially [ɪ'speʃəli] *adv.* 尤其，特别是　*e.g.* especially when 尤其是……的时候

practice ['præktɪs] *n.* 练习　*e.g.* yoga practice 瑜伽练习

before bed 睡觉之前

adrenal gland 肾上腺

2.3.6　青蛙式

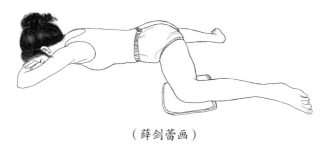

（薛剑蕾画）

◆无论我们在哪里，我们都要学会恰当地处理事情。

Step-by-step Instructions

Be on your hands and knees with your palms under your shoulders and your knees under your hips.

Rest your forearms on the floor with your elbows directly under your shoulders.

Walk your knees out to the sides one at a time to open your hips, slowly lowering your torso. Put a folded blanket under your knees as needed to provide cushioning.

Align your thighs and lower legs to a 90-degree angle and flex your ankles.

Walk your elbows forward with your upper arms and forearms forming a 90-degree angle. Spread your fingers wide apart for support.

To release more deeply into the pose, press your lower legs and feet downward, holding for a count of five, and then release, walking your knees a little farther out. Repeat this action several times, then hold the pose.

If comfortable, move into full Frog pose by lowering your chest to the floor and resting your forehead on the back of your hands with the right hand on top of your left or the other way around.

Benefits

Frog pose can help

· improve posture

· stimulate abdominal organs

· improve blood circulation in the pelvic region

· improve flexibility in the hip joints and inner thighs

· stretch the ankles, inner thighs, groin, abdomen and hip flexors

◆ A family life is a training place for public life. If you can't face a sharp word from your mate, how can you face such words from a stranger?

步骤说明

双手双膝支撑，手掌在肩膀下方，双膝在髋部下方。

小臂放于地板上，肘部在肩膀正下方。

双膝逐一向外侧移动以打开髋部，躯干慢慢落下来。根据需要，在双膝下方放一个折叠的毯子以提供缓冲。

调整大腿与小腿成90度角，勾脚踝。

手肘向前移动，保持大臂与小臂成90度角。手指大大地分开以提供支撑。

要更深入体式，小腿和双脚向下压，数5个数，然后放松，双膝再向外移动一点。将这个动作重复几次，然后保持住。

如果感觉舒适的话，可以让胸部落在地板上，右手叠放在左手上或反过来左手在上，额头放在手背上，进入完全青蛙式。

益处

青蛙式能够帮助

· 改善体态

· 刺激腹部器官

· 促进骨盆区域血液循环

· 提高髋关节和大腿内侧灵活度

· 拉伸脚踝、大腿内侧、腹股沟、腹部及髋部屈肌

◆家庭生活是公共生活的训练场。如果你无法面对伴侣的尖锐言辞，你又怎能面对陌生人的尖锐言辞呢?

Contraindications and Cautions

Don't practise Frog pose if you have hernia. Practise with one knee bent at a time and with a cushion under the knees in case of hip, knee or ankle issues.

Words and Expressions / 词汇表达

frog [frɒg] *n.* 青蛙

provide [prə'vaɪd] *v.* 提供 ***e.g.*** provide service 提供服务

cushion ['kʊʃn] *v.* 起缓冲作用，缓和冲击 ***e.g.*** cushion the blow 减轻打击

more [mɔː] *adv.* 更多，此外，更大程度地 ***e.g.*** more accurate 更准确

count [kaʊnt] *n.* 数数，点数 ***e.g.*** a count of 8 数到8

a little 一点儿

◆ The world is a training place where we learn to use the world without getting attached.

禁忌和注意事项

如果你有疝气，不要练习青蛙式。如果髋部、膝盖或脚踝有问题，每次练习时单侧屈膝，并在膝下垫一个垫子。

farther ['fɑːðə] *adv.* 更远地，更进一步地　*e.g.* jump farther 跳得更远

time [taɪm] *n.* 次，回　*e.g.* next time 下一次

move into 进入

the other way around 反过来，倒过来

hip flexor [hɪp]['fleksə] *n.* 髋屈肌

cushion ['kʊʃn] *n.* 软垫，坐垫　*e.g.* a floor cushion 地板坐垫

issue ['ɪʃuː] *n.* 问题　*e.g.* health issue 健康问题

◆世界是一个训练场，我们在这里学习如何利用而不依附这个世界。

2.4 Supine Poses

2.4.1 Viparīta Karaṇī / Legs-up-the-wall pose[7]

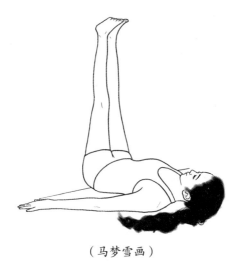

（马梦雪画）

Step-by-step Instructions

Sitting sideways next to a wall, slowly recline onto your back while swiveling your hips toward the wall and extending both legs up the wall.

Adjust your legs so that they are perpendicular to the floor. If your hamstrings are too tight to do so, slide your hips out away from the wall.

You may place a folded blanket under your lower back for support or hold your legs together with a strap and place a sandbag on your feet

---

◆ The same world can be a heaven or a hell.

2.4 仰卧体式

2.4.1 靠墙倒剪式⑦

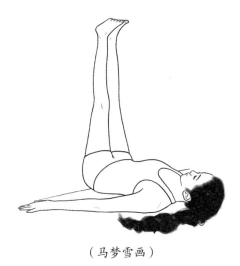

（马梦雪画）

步骤说明

靠墙侧坐，臀部转向墙面的同时慢慢仰卧下来，双腿在墙面
伸展向上。

调整双腿与地板垂直。如果腘绳肌太紧无法做到，滑动臀部
向外离开墙壁。

你可以将折叠的毯子放在下背部下方用来支撑，或者用伸展

◆同一个世界可以是天堂，也可以是地狱。

for stability.

You can rest your palms on the belly and heart, or drape your arms onto the floor with palms facing up.

Stay in this position for as long as is comfortable with normal breathing.

To come down, bend your knees and roll to the right side and sit up.

Benefits

Legs-up-the-wall pose can help

· regulate blood pressure

· alleviate menstrual disorders, palpitations, breathlessness and asthma

· relieve indigestion, diarrhea, nausea and lower back pain

· reduce soreness or inflammation in the abdominal area

Contraindications and Cautions

Avoid practising this pose during menstruation.

Words and Expressions / 词汇表达

sideways ['saɪdweɪz] *adv.* 向侧面地，向一旁地 *e.g.* look sideways 斜视

next to 紧挨着

recline [rɪ'klaɪn] *v.* 向后倚靠 *e.g.* recline on a sofa 靠在沙发上

swivel ['swɪvl] *v.* 转身，转动 *e.g.* swivel around 转过来

adjust [ə'dʒʌst] *v.* 调整，调节 *e.g.* adjust price 调整价格

◆ Before you learn to swim, water seems to be a dreadful place. But once you learn to swim, you will love the water.

带将双腿绑在一起，并在脚上放置沙袋以保持稳定。

手掌可停留在腹部和心脏处，或者双臂搭放在地板上，掌心朝上。

保持正常呼吸，在舒适的状态下保持这个体式。

下来时，屈膝滚动到右侧然后坐立起身。

益处

靠墙倒剪式能够帮助

· 调节血压

· 缓解月经紊乱、心悸、呼吸困难和哮喘

· 缓解消化不良、腹泻、恶心和下背部疼痛

· 减少腹部的疼痛或炎症

禁忌和注意事项

经期避免练习这个体式。

---

too...to... 太……以至不能

tight [taɪt] *adj.* 紧的，紧绷的　*e.g.* tight muscles 僵紧的肌肉

stability [stə'bɪləti] *n.* 稳定，稳定性　*e.g.* emotional stability 情绪的稳定性

drape [dreɪp] *v.* 搭在，垂下　*e.g.* drape...around... 使（身体部位）轻松地搭在……上

◆在你学会游泳之前，水域似乎是一个可怕的地方。但是一旦你学会游泳，你就会爱上水。

come down 下来

roll [rəʊl] *v.* 滚动，翻身　*e.g.* roll into 滚进

2.4.2　Ānanda Bālāsana / Happy Baby pose

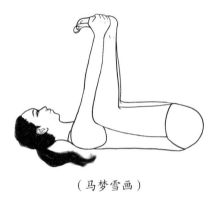

（马梦雪画）

Step-by-step Instructions

Lie on your back. Raise both arms and legs into the air and loosen them by shaking them gently. Stop shaking and hold your arms and legs upward.

Inhale, catch hold of the outsides of your feet with your hands (If you have difficulty doing so, grip your ankles or hold onto a strap looped over each sole).

Open your knees and bring them up toward your armpits. Position your ankles directly over the knees so that your shins are perpendicular to the floor. Check that the soles of your feet face the ceiling.

◆ Anything we call ours cannot be ours.

regulate ['regjuleɪt] *v.* 调节　***e.g.*** regulate the flow of water 调节水流
pain [peɪn] *n.* 疼痛　***e.g.*** relieve the pain in... 缓解（某部位）的疼痛

2.4.2　快乐婴儿式

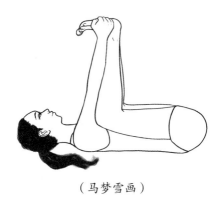

（马梦雪画）

步骤说明

仰卧。双臂和双腿抬向空中，轻轻抖动以放松。停止抖动，手臂和双腿保持上举。

吸气，双手抓住双脚的外侧（如果这样做有困难，那就抓住你的脚踝或者抓住圈套在每只脚上的伸展带）。

打开双膝并将它们向上拉向腋窝。脚踝置于膝盖的正上方，让小腿胫骨垂直于地板。确保脚掌朝向天花板。

◆一切我们称为我们的都不可能是我们的。

Pull your hands down to draw your knees closer to your armpits while your head and shoulders rest on the floor.

Remain in this pose for as long as is comfortable with natural breathing.

To come out of the pose, release your feet, rest your arms and legs on the floor and relax.

Benefits

Happy Baby pose can help
· stretch the spine and inner groin
· calm the brain and relieve stress and fatigue

Contraindications and Cautions

Don't practise this pose in case of pregnancy or knee injury. People with neck injury should support the head on a thickly folded blanket.

Words and Expressions / 词汇表达

happy ['hæpi] *adj.* 高兴的，快乐的，幸福的　*e.g.* a happy family 一个幸福的家庭

baby ['beɪbi] *n.* 婴儿　*e.g.* baby boom 婴儿潮

both...and... 两者都

air [eə] *n.* 空中，天空　*e.g.* in the air 在空中

shake [ʃeɪk] *v.* 摇动，晃动　*e.g.* shake hands 握手

stop doing 停止做……

◆ We speak ourselves in two ways. One is, "Look at my body. Isn't it slim?" The other is, "Look at how slim I am." Who is slim? Is it you or the body? This identification with other things is the cause of all our pain.

保持头部和肩膀停留在地板上，双手向下拉让双膝更靠近腋窝。

保持自然呼吸，在舒适的状态下保持这个体式。

退出体式时，松开双脚，手臂和双腿停留在地板上，放松。

益处

快乐婴儿式能够帮助

·伸展脊柱及腹股沟内侧

·让大脑平静并缓解压力与疲劳

禁忌和注意事项

如果处于孕期或膝盖受伤，不要练习这个体式。颈部受伤的人应该将毯子厚厚地折叠起来支撑头部。

the outside of the foot 脚外侧

loop [luːp] v. 使成环，使绕成圈　*e.g.* loop around 打环套在……上

check [tʃek] v. 查看，核实，确保　*e.g.* check with somebody 与某人核实

natural ['nætʃrəl] *adj.* 自然的　*e.g.* natural reaction 自然反应

support [sə'pɔːt] v. 支撑　*e.g.* be supported by 由……所支撑

thickly ['θɪkli] *adv.* 厚厚地　*e.g.* dress thickly 穿得厚厚地

◆我们用两种方式表达自己。一种是，"看看我的身体。是不是很苗条呀？"另一种是，"看看我有多苗条。"谁苗条？是你还是你的身体？这种与其他事物等同起来的做法是我们所有痛苦的根源。

2.4.3 Pāvānamuktāsana / Wind-relieving pose

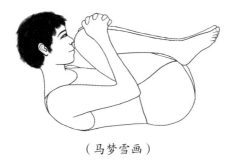

(马梦雪画)

Step-by-step Instructions

Lie on your back with your legs and feet together, hands alongside your body.

Bend your right knee, interlock the fingers and clasp your hands on the shin, pressing the thigh towards your chest. Keep your left leg straight on the floor.

Inhale deeply. Exhale, raise your shoulders and head up and try to touch your right knee with your nose. Relax your neck, shoulders and abdomen.

Maintain this pose for a few more deep breaths.

Inhale, lower your shoulders and head back to the floor. Exhale, release your right leg and relax. Repeat with your left leg.

Bend both knees, interlock the fingers and clasp your hands on the shinbones, bringing the thighs close to your chest.

Take a deep breath. Exhale, raise your shoulders and head, relax your shoulders down and try to place your nose in the space between the two knees.

◆ If something changes, we should let it go — something else will come. We should watch the changes like watching passing clouds.

2.4.3　排气式

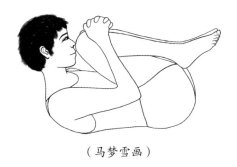

（马梦雪画）

步骤说明

仰卧，双腿双脚并拢，双手置于身体两侧。

屈右膝，十指交扣，双手紧抱小腿胫骨，将大腿压向胸部。保持左腿在地板上伸直。

深长地吸气。呼气，肩膀和头部向上抬起，尽量让鼻子触碰右膝。颈部、肩膀和腹部放松。

保持这个姿势再做几次深呼吸。

吸气，肩膀和头部落回地面。呼气，松开右腿，放松。换左腿重复上述动作。

屈双膝，十指交扣，双手环抱小腿胫骨，将大腿拉近胸部。

深吸一口气。呼气，肩膀和头部抬起，双肩放松下沉，尽量将鼻子置于双膝之间。

◆如果有些事情发生了变化，我们应该随它去——还有别的会来。我们应该像观看浮云一般来看待这些变化。

Hold this position for as long as is comfortable while retaining the breath.

Inhale, slowly lower your shoulders and head back to the floor. Exhale, straighten your legs and relax.

Benefits

Wind-relieving pose can help

· remove stiffness in the neck, knees, hips and buttocks

· strengthen the lower back muscles

· massage the abdomen and digestive organs and therefore is effective in removing wind, indigestion and constipation

Contraindications and Cautions

This pose should be avoided by people with high blood pressure or serious back problems such as sciatica and slipped disc.

Words and Expressions / 词汇表达

wind [wɪnd] *n.* 胃气, 肠气　*e.g.* break wind 放屁

alongside [ə͵lɒŋ'saɪd] *prep.* 在……旁边　*e.g.* arms alongside the body 双臂放身体两侧

a few more 再多几个

digestive organ 消化器官

◆ Changes are like flowing water. If you just allow water to flow, it is very pleasant to sit and watch. But if you want to arrest the flow and keep the water for yourself, you will have to construct a dam. Then the water will resist the dam and try to escape. There will be a terrible struggle.

保持呼吸，在舒适的状态下保持这个体式。

吸气，肩膀和头部慢慢落回到地板上。呼气，伸直双腿，放松。

益处

排气式能够帮助

· 消除颈部、膝盖、髋部及臀部的僵硬感

· 强健下背部肌肉

· 按摩腹部和消化器官，因此能有效地排气、消食和通便

禁忌和注意事项

有高血压或严重的背部问题，如坐骨神经痛和椎间盘突出，应避免这个体式。

---

therefore ['ðeəfɔ:] *adv.* 因此，所以

effective [ɪ'fektɪv] *adj.* 有效的，起作用的　　*e.g.* effective measures 有效措施

such as 例如，比如

◆变化犹如流水。如果你任水流动，坐而观之是非常愉快的。但如果你想要阻止水流，留给自己，你就必须建造水坝。然后水会抵抗大坝并试图逃跑。必将有一番可怕的争斗。

2.4.4　Halāsana / Plow pose

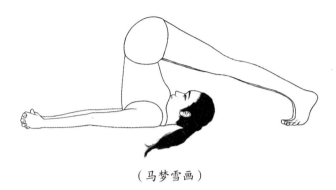

（马梦雪画）

Step-by-step Instructions

Lie flat on your back, and align your head, neck and spine. Keep your legs stretched out and place your arms alongside your body, palms down.

Please bear in mind that you don't sneeze, cough or clear your throat while in the pose, or turn your head from side to side.

Inhale, with your knees straight, raise your legs to a 90-degree angle. Exhale, press on your palms, contract your pelvic floor and abdominal muscles to raise your legs straight up and bring your hands immediately to support your back.

See that your trunk is perpendicular to the floor and your chest touches the chin. Rest your elbows on the floor.

Exhale, slowly move your legs overhead and lower your toes onto the floor. Keep your thighs active by pulling your kneecaps up.

You may keep your hands on your back for support, stretch your arms on the floor in the direction opposite to that of the legs, or clasp your hands and press your arms actively down on the floor.

◆ All life is a passing show. If we want to hold it, even for a minute, we will feel tension.

2.4.4　犁式

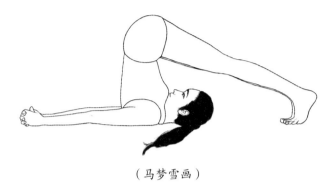

（马梦雪画）

步骤说明

平躺下来，头部、颈部及脊柱对齐。保持双腿向外伸展，双臂置于身体两侧，掌心向下。

请记住，在这个体式中不要打喷嚏、咳嗽或清嗓子，头部也不要左右转动。

吸气，保持双膝伸直，双腿抬高成90度角。呼气，手掌下压，收缩骨盆底和腹肌，将双腿直接抬起并立即用手支撑背部。

确保躯干垂直于地板，胸触下巴。手肘停放在地板上。

呼气，慢慢地将双腿移过头顶，脚趾落在地板上。通过髋骨上提保持大腿处于激活状态。

你可以保持双手在背部支撑，手臂在地板上向双腿相反的方向伸展，或双手扣紧，手臂主动压向地板。

◆所有的生命都是一场短暂的演出。如果我们想抓住它，哪怕只有一分钟，我们都会感到紧张。

Remain in this pose for 20 to 30 seconds with normal breathing.

To come out of the pose, with hands on your back for support, bend your knees and slowly roll down onto your back with an exhalation. Extend your legs, place your palms by the sides, and relax.

Benefits

Plow pose can help

· relieve headache, backache, lumbago, fatigue, and stiff shoulders and elbows

· stimulate the abdominal organs and the thyroid gland

· soothe the brain and the nerves

· relieve the symptoms of menstrual and urinary system disorders

Contraindications and Cautions

Avoid this pose during menstruation or if you have a neck injury, shoulder problem or diarrhea.

Words and Expressions / 词汇表达

plow [plaʊ] *n.* 犁

bear in mind 记住，牢记在心

sneeze [sni:z] *v.* 打喷嚏　*e.g.* sneeze loudly 大声打喷嚏

cough [kɒf] *v.* 咳嗽　*e.g.* cough violently 剧烈地咳嗽

clear one's throat 清清嗓子

from side to side 从一边到另一边，左右（摇摆）

immediately [ɪ'mi:dɪətlɪ] *adv.* 立即，直接地　*e.g.* immediately disappear 立即消失

◆ As long as we learn to enjoy each change, we can recognize the beauty even in aging.

在这个体式中保持20到30秒，正常呼吸。

退出体式时，双手于背部支撑，随着呼气，屈膝，慢慢滚动仰卧下来。双腿伸展，手掌置于身体两侧，放松。

益处

犁式能够帮助

· 缓解头痛、背痛、腰痛、疲劳以及肩肘僵硬

· 刺激腹部器官和甲状腺

· 舒缓大脑和神经

· 缓解月经和泌尿系统紊乱的症状

禁忌和注意事项

经期或者颈部受伤、肩膀有问题、腹泻，避免练习该体式。

---

pelvic floor 骨盆底

active ['æktɪv] *adj.* 活跃的，起作用的 *e.g.* an active volcano 一座活火山

direction [dɪ'rekʃn] *n.* 方向 *e.g.* in the direction of 朝……的方向

opposite to 与……相反，在……对面

actively ['æktɪvli] *adv.* 主动地，积极地 *e.g.* actively look for a job 积极地找工作

thyroid gland 甲状腺

◆只要我们学会享受每一个变化，我们甚至能在衰老中发现美。

2.4.5   Supta Vīrāsana / Reclining Hero pose

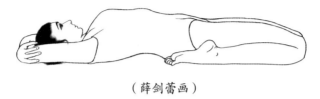

（薛剑蕾画）

Step-by-step Instructions

Kneel on the floor (use a folded blanket to wedge between your calves and thighs if necessary), with your thighs perpendicular to the floor, and touch your inner knees together.

Slide your feet apart, slightly wider than your hips. Turn your soles toward the ceiling. Each of your toes should rest on the floor. Adjust your legs by turning in your thighs and turning out your calves.

Then sit down between your feet. Make sure both sitting bones are evenly supported.

Place your hands on the floor behind your toes, shoulder-width apart with your fingers pointing toward the toes. Your torso naturally inclines backward.

Exhale, lower your back gradually toward the floor. Rest your elbows, one by one, on the floor.

Make sure that both your shoulder blades remain flat on the floor and do not let your buttocks or knees lift off the floor. Release your back and allow it to descend completely to the floor (Put a long bolster lengthwise behind your back as needed and rest your spine evenly on it).

◆ When we just allow things to pass, we are free. Things will just come and go while we retain our peace.

2.4.5　仰卧英雄式

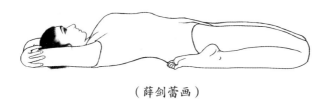

（薛剑蕾画）

步骤说明

跪立于地板上（如果必要的话，使用折叠的毯子塞进小腿肚与大腿之间），大腿垂直于地板，双膝内缘相触。

双脚滑动分开，略宽于髋部。脚心转动朝向天花板。每一根脚趾都应贴地。调整双腿，大腿内旋，小腿肚外旋。

然后，坐于双脚之间。确保两侧坐骨均匀地被支撑。

双手放于脚趾后方的地板上，打开与肩同宽，手指冲向脚趾。躯干自然向后倾斜。

呼气，后背逐步落向地板。手肘逐一停放到地板上。

确保两侧肩胛骨在地板上放平，不要让臀部或膝盖抬离地板。放松背部，让它完全沉落到地板上（根据需要，把一个长型抱枕纵向放在背后，让脊柱均匀地停放在上面）。

◆当我们任由事情过去，我们就是自由的。事情来来去去，我们保有平和。

Extend your arms out to the sides with your palms facing up. Explore drawing your arms overhead and clasping the elbows.

Breathe evenly and stay in this pose for 20 to 30 seconds.

To come out, press your forearms against the floor and come onto your hands. As you come up, lead with your sternum, not your head or chin.

Benefits

Reclining Hero pose can help

· stretch the abdomen, the back and the waist

· lengthen the psoas and the deep inner muscles

· relieve acidity, heartburn, stomachache, back pain, and menstrual cramps

· relax the nerves, diaphragm, and the abdominal muscles

· improve flexibility of the knees and ankles

· remove tiredness in the legs

Contraindications and Cautions

Don't practise this pose if you have lumbar lordosis, severe arthritis of the hip, knee or ankle, a torn meniscus, or a recent abdominal or breast incision, or a hernia. Avoid this pose during menstruation.

◆ The more we enjoy, the more we are bound. While enjoying, we are not going to listen to wisdom unless we have extraordinary intelligence.

手臂向两侧伸展，掌心向上。试探着将双臂举过头顶，互抱手肘。

均匀地呼吸，在这个体式中停留20到30秒。

退出时，小臂下压地板，然后双手支撑。起来时，用你的胸骨而非头或下巴引领起身。

益处

仰卧英雄式能够帮助

·拉伸腹部、背部及腰部

·拉长腰肌和深层内肌

·缓解胃酸过多、胃灼热、胃痛、背痛和痛经

·放松神经、横隔膜和腹部肌肉

·提升膝盖和脚踝的灵活性

·消除腿部疲劳

禁忌和注意事项

如果你有腰椎前凸，严重的髋、膝、踝关节炎，半月板撕裂，或近期有腹部、乳腺切口抑或疝气，不要练习这个体式。在经期时避免这个体式。

◆我们享受得越多，受的束缚就越多。在享受的时候，我们不会去聆听智慧，除非我们有非凡的才智。

Words and Expressions / 词汇表达

reclining [rɪ'klaɪnɪŋ] *adj.* 倾斜的，向后倚靠的　*e.g.* reclining chair 躺椅

hero ['hɪərəʊ] *n.* 英雄　*e.g.* a real hero 一个真正的英雄

kneel [ni:l] *v.* 跪下　*e.g.* kneel down 跪下

wedge [wedʒ] *v.* 将……挤入（或塞进，插入）　*e.g.* wedge...into 将……塞入，挤进

sit down 坐下

naturally ['nætʃrəli] *adv.* 自然地　*e.g.* breathe naturally 自然地呼吸

2.4.6　Śavāsana / Corpse pose

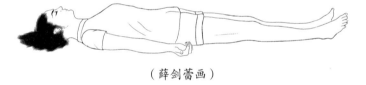

（薛剑蕾画）

Step-by-step Instructions

Lie on your back with your knees bent and the soles of your feet on the floor.

Gently engage the bandha[8] and lift your hips off the earth, tucking your tailbone in. Lower your spine one vertebra at a time, creating length along your entire spinal column.

Lift your chest a little to let your shoulder blades relax slightly toward each other, then lie back down with more spaciousness across your heart centre.

◆ The very word "understand" is a combination of two words: "under" and "stand." To understand, we should stand under. Under where we now stand.

incline [ɪn'klaɪn] *v.* （使）倾斜　***e.g.*** incline towards 朝……倾斜

one by one 一个接一个，逐一

flat [flæt] *adj.* 平的，平坦的　***e.g.*** flat surface 平面

explore [ɪk'splɔː] *v.* （用手或身体某部位）探查，探索　***e.g.*** try to explore 努力去探索

lead [liːd] *v.* 引领　***e.g.*** lead the way 领路

recent ['riːsnt] *adj.* 最近的，近期的　***e.g.*** in recent years 在近几年

incision [ɪn'sɪʒn] *n.* 切口　***e.g.*** horizontal incision 水平切口

2.4.6　挺尸式

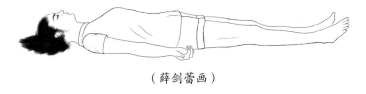

（薛剑蕾画）

步骤说明

仰卧并屈膝，脚掌踩地。

轻柔地启用能量锁⑧，臀部抬离地面，尾骨内收。让脊柱逐节放下，沿着整根脊柱拉长。

胸抬起一点，两侧肩胛骨微微放松靠拢，让心脏中心处有更多的空间感，然后再躺回去。

◆ "Understand"（理解）这个词由两个词组成：under（在……之下）和 stand（站立）。要理解，我们就得站在下面。站在我们现在所站之处的下面。

Straighten your legs one at a time with your feet separated slightly wider than your hips, allowing your feet to naturally turn outward.

Rest your arms and hands at a comfortable distance from your torso. Turn your palms to face the ceiling.

Tuck your chin slightly in to lengthen your neck with your forehead parallel to the floor. Make sure that the centre part of the back of your head rests on the floor. If your head is thrown back, you may put a folded blanket under your head.

Let loose your body. Feel as though your body is completely dropped onto the floor.

Keep your eyes closed and focus on your deep breathing, feeling the simple rising and falling of your chest and belly.

Take one last deep inhalation, then with the exhalation, let everything go, allowing your breath to flow however it naturally will.

Stay in Corpse pose for at least five minutes.

Benefits

Corpse pose can help

· remove physical and mental fatigue and therefore one can practise it whenever one feels physically and mentally tired

· relieve migraines, stress-induced headaches, insomnia and high blood pressure

· soothe the nervous system and calm the mind

· develop awareness of the body

◆ We should know where we stand first and then try to "under" stand, to go a little deeper.

逐一伸直双腿。双脚打开略宽于髋部，让双脚自然外展。

让双臂和双手在躯干两侧舒适的距离处停留。掌心转动朝向天花板。

微收下巴以拉长颈部，前额与地面平行。确保后脑勺中部贴地。如果头部后仰，可以在头部下方垫一个折叠的毯子。

释放掉你的身体。感觉身体好像完全地瘫在地板上。

保持双眼闭合，把注意力放到深呼吸上，单纯去感受胸腔和腹部的起起伏伏。

最后一次深吸气，然后随着呼气，放开一切，让你的呼吸自然地流动。

在挺尸式中停留至少5分钟。

益处

挺尸式能够帮助

·消除身心疲劳，因此无论何时感到身心疲惫都可以练习这个体式

·缓解偏头痛、压力引起的头痛、失眠以及高血压

·舒缓神经系统，使头脑平静

·培养对身体的意识

◆我们应该先知道自己所处的位置，然后试着站到"下面"，再深入一点。

Contraindications and Cautions

In case of pregnancy, anxiety or respiratory ailment, prastice Corpse pose with the head and chest supported on a bolster. Do not move the body at all during the practice.

Words and Expressions / 词汇表达

corpse [kɔːps] *n.* 尸体　　***e.g.*** a corpse 一具尸体

spinal column 脊柱

more [mɔː] *adj.* 更多的　　***e.g.*** more time 更多的时间

spaciousness ['speɪʃəsnɪs] *n.* 宽敞，宽广　　***e.g.*** a feeling of spaciousness 一种宽敞的感觉

outward ['aʊtwəd] *adv.* 向外（同 outwards）　　***e.g.*** move outward 向外移动

at [æt] *prep.* 从相隔……远的地方　　***e.g.*** at a distance of... ……之远；相距

from [frɒm] *prep.*（表示两地的距离）离　　***e.g.*** far away from 远离

the back of the head 脑后，后脑勺

throw [θrəʊ] *v.* 猛动（身体或身体部位），仰起（头）　　***e.g.*** throw oneself onto the bed 一头倒在床上

let loose 让……自由，释放，放开

as though 好像，仿佛

drop [drɒp] *v.*（身体部位无力地）垂下，使落下　　***e.g.*** drop into a chair 瘫坐在椅子上

simple ['sɪmpl] *adj.* 纯粹的，完全的　　***e.g.*** a simple truth 纯粹的事实

◆ When we try to understand, we will find we are not all on one "stand" but at different levels, with different capacities, tastes and temperaments.

禁忌和注意事项

如果处于孕期、焦虑或有呼吸系统疾病，练习挺尸式时将头和胸部支撑在瑜伽抱枕上。练习过程中身体不要移动。

rising and falling 升降，起伏

last [lɑːst] *adj.* 最后的　***e.g.*** the last train 末班车

let go 放开，释放

flow [fləʊ] *v.*（液体，气体或电）流动　***e.g.*** flow slowly 缓慢地流动

will [wɪl] *v.* 愿意，想要　***e.g.*** if you will 如果你愿意的话

at least 至少

minute ['mɪnɪt] *n.* 分钟，片刻　***e.g.*** several minutes 几分钟

physical ['fɪzɪkl] *adj.* 身体的　***e.g.*** physical health 身体健康

mental ['mentl] *adj.* 精神的，脑力的，心理上的　***e.g.*** mental age 心理年龄

physically ['fɪzɪkli] *adv.* 肉体上，身体上　***e.g.*** physically strong 身体强壮的

mentally ['mentəli] *adv.* 精神上，智力上，心理上　***e.g.*** mentally disturbed 心理不正常

tired ['taɪəd] *adj.* 疲倦的　***e.g.*** dog tired 累趴下

induce [ɪn'djuːs] *v.* 引起，导致　***e.g.*** drug-induced abortion 药物流产

develop [dɪ'veləp] *v.* 养成　***e.g.*** develop a habit 养成习惯

◆当我们试着去理解的时候，我们会发现我们并非都站在同一个"立场"上，而是处在不同的层次上，有着不同的能力、品味和性情。

2.5　Other Frequently-seen Yoga Poses

2.5.1　Mārjāriāsana / Cat Stretch pose⑨

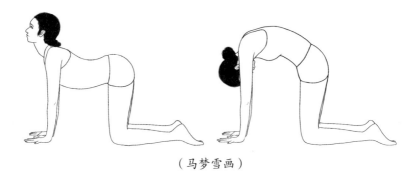

（马梦雪画）

Step-by-step Instructions

Come onto your hands and knees, with your knees directly below your hips and your hands below your shoulders.

Make sure your hands are flat on the floor with the fingers pointing forward. The tops of your feet rest on the floor. Your arms and legs are perpendicular to the floor and parallel to each other.

As you inhale, raise the tailbone up, concave your back, lift your chin and head and look up. Feel that your chest expands and the front of your neck elongates.

As you exhale, roll the tailbone down, arch your back upward, lower your head and draw your chin towards the chest.

◆ The world is our factory. As we pass through we are shaped every minute by different experiences. We become refined as our knowledge develops.

2.5　其他常见瑜伽体式

2.5.1　猫伸展式[9]

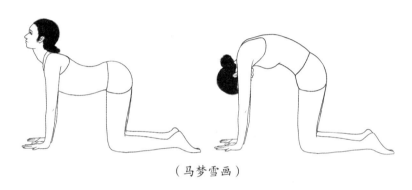

（马梦雪画）

步骤说明

双手和双膝着地，双膝在臀部正下方，双手在肩膀正下方。

确保双手平放在地板上，手指指向前方。脚背贴地。双臂和双腿垂直于地板且相互平行。

随着吸气，尾骨上提，背部下凹，下巴与头部上抬，向上看。感受胸腔扩张，颈部前侧拉长。

随着呼气，卷尾骨向下，背部向上弓起，低头，下巴拉近胸部。

◆世界是我们的加工厂。当我们经过时，每一分钟都被不同的经历所塑造。随着知识的增长，我们变得更有教养。

(Inhale into cow position and exhale into cat position.) Continue for a few more rounds at your own pace. See that each movement coordinates with your breath.

Benefits

Cat stretch pose can help

· improve flexibility of the neck, shoulders and spine

· strengthen the muscles of the back and relieve back pain and tension

· tone the female reproductive system and relieve menstrual cramps

Contraindications and Cautions

Be careful with the way you distribute your weight on your hands. Spread your fingers and press with your palms instead of putting all the pressure on the heels of the hands.

Words and Expressions / 词汇表达

cat [kæt] *n.* 猫

concave [kɒn'keɪv] *v.* 使变凹形　*e.g.* concave one's belly 腹部向内凹

arch [ɑːtʃ] *v.* （使）弯成弓形　*e.g.* arch your back 弓背

round [raʊnd] *n.* 轮次，回合　*e.g.* a round of（运动比赛等的）一轮；一场

at one's own pace 以某人自己的节奏

movement ['muːvmənt] *n.* （身体部位的）运动，动作　*e.g.* body

◆ Once I thought all these were real: money, name, position, beauty. But now I understand that none of these is permanent. When that understanding comes, we no longer trust the worldly pleasures nor run after them.

（吸气进入牛式，呼气进入猫式。）以你自己的节奏继续做几组。确保每个动作都配合你的呼吸来做。

益处

猫伸展式能够帮助

·提升颈部、肩部和脊柱的灵活性

·强健背部肌肉，缓解背部疼痛和紧张

·调理女性生殖系统，缓解痛经

禁忌和注意事项

注意将身体重量分布在手上的方式。手指分开，用你的手掌按压，而不是把所有的压力放在掌根。

movement 肢体动作

coordinate with 使与……协调，配合

female ['fiːmeɪl] *adj.* 女性的　*e.g.* a female teacher 一位女老师

way [weɪ] *n.* 方式，方法　*e.g.* in this way 以这样的方式

instead of 而不是

pressure ['preʃə] *n.* 压力　*e.g.* under pressure 在压力之下，承受压力

the heel of the hand 掌根

◆曾经我以为这一切都是真实的：金钱、名声、地位、美貌。但现在我明白了，这一切都不是永恒的。当有了这种理解时，我们不再相信世俗的享乐，也不再追求它们。

2.5.2 Adho Mukha Śvānāsana / Downward-facing Dog pose

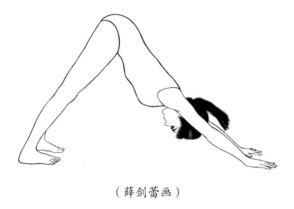

（薛剑蕾画）

Step-by-step Instructions

Come onto your hands and knees, with toes tucked under. Check that your knees are directly below your hips and your hands are slightly in front of your shoulders. Spread your fingers widely.

Inhale deeply. Exhale, pressing down evenly through your fingers and palms, lift your knees off the floor.

Shift your weight backward, extend your arms away from your hands, and tuck your shoulder blades in to broaden your chest. Your abdomen should be contracted and hips lifted.

See that your spine is lengthened and your back is fully extended. Your head and neck should be in alignment with your spine.

Walk your heels one at a time to lengthen the back of your legs. Keep your legs straight, lift your kneecaps and sitting bones and push

---

◆ Escapism never helps us. If we try to leave something now, we will have to face it in a more difficult form later on.

2.5.2　下犬式

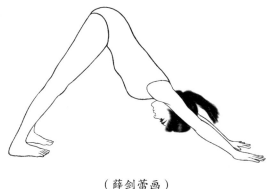

（薛剑蕾画）

步骤说明

双手和双膝着地，脚趾踮地。确保双膝在臀部正下方，双手位置比肩膀稍往前一点。手指大大地分开。

深吸气。呼气，手指和手掌均匀地向下压，双膝抬离地面。

将你的身体重心后移，手臂伸展远离双手，肩胛骨内收，扩展胸腔。腹部收紧，臀部上提。

确保脊柱拉长，背部完全展开。你的头部和颈部应该与脊柱在一条直线上。

脚跟逐一上下踩动拉长腿部后侧。保持双腿伸直，髌骨与坐骨上提，大腿向后推。

◆逃避现实对我们毫无帮助。如果我们现在试图留下一些东西，我们之后将不得不以一种更为困难的形式面对它。

your thighs back.

Lower your heels toward the floor. Keep your feet parallel to each other and extend the toes.

Hold this pose for 20 to 30 seconds with deep breathing.

To come out of the pose, lower your knees to the floor, press your hips back towards your heels and relax.

Benefits

Downward-facing Dog pose can help

· calm the brain and restore energy

· stimulate the nervous system

· strengthen the wrists, arms, legs and ankles

· stretch the hands, shoulders, hamstrings, calves, and arches

· reduce stiffness in the heels and shoulders

· relieve stress, mild depression, headache, insomnia, back discomfort and fatigue

Contraindications and Cautions

Avoid this pose if you are in an advanced stage of pregnancy or if you have diarrhea. If you have high blood pressure or headache, you can choose to support your head on a bolster or block. If you have wrist problems, talk to your doctor first. In this pose, you have to be sure it is more important to keep the back straight than to keep the legs straight.

◆ The answer is the same, but the method of working it out may vary this way or that.

脚跟落向地板。保持双脚互相平行，脚趾伸展。

伴随深长的呼吸，在这个体式中停留20到30秒。

退出体式时，双膝落到地板上，臀部向后压向脚跟，放松。

益处

下犬式能够帮助

- 让大脑平静并恢复能量
- 刺激神经系统
- 强健手腕、手臂、双腿和脚踝
- 伸展手、肩膀、腘绳肌、小腿肚和足弓
- 减少脚跟和肩膀的僵硬感
- 缓解压力、轻度抑郁、头痛、失眠、背部不适及疲劳

禁忌和注意事项

如果处于妊娠晚期或者有腹泻，避免这个体式。如果有高血压或头痛，可以选择用抱枕或瑜伽砖支撑头部。如果手腕有问题，请先咨询医生。在这个体式中，你必须确信保持背部平直比保持双腿伸直更为重要。

◆答案是一样的，但是计算出它的方法可能有这样或那样的不同。

Words and Expressions / 词汇表达

under ['ʌndə] *adv.* 在下面　*e.g.* go under 沉没

forward ['fɔːrwərd] *adj.* 向前的　*e.g.* forward movement 前进，向前移动

widely ['waɪdli] *adv.* 大大地，很大程度上　*e.g.* vary widely 千差万别

broaden ['brɔːdn] *v.* 使扩大，使变宽　*e.g.* broaden out 加宽（路，河等）

fully ['fʊli] *adv.* 充分地，完全地　*e.g.* fully understand 完全理解

in alignment with 与⋯⋯成一直线

push [pʊʃ] *v.* 推　*e.g.* push away 推开

2.5.3　Ardha Matsyendrāsana / Half Lord-of-the-fish pose

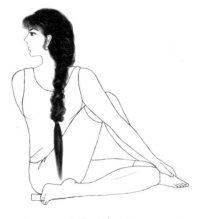

（薛剑蕾画）

◆ Every experience in the world is mental. We might put our minds onto something and think, "This is really great", but once our attention goes somewhere else, that thing becomes nothing to us.

restore [rɪ'stɔː] *v.* 恢复，使复原　***e.g.*** restore order 恢复秩序

energy ['enədʒi] *n.* 能量，精力　***e.g.*** energy field 能量场

advanced stage 晚期

choose to 选择

talk to 与……谈话

It is more...to do...than to do... 做……比做……更……

important [ɪm'pɔːtnt] *adj.* 重要的　***e.g.*** an important meeting 一个重要
的会议

2.5.3　半鱼王式

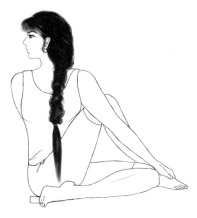

（薛剑蕾画）

◆世界上的每一种体验都是心灵层面的。我们可能会把注意力放在某件
事情上，然后想，"这真的太棒了"，但是一旦我们的注意力转移到其他地
方，那件事对我们来说就什么都不是了。

Step-by-step Instructions

Sit in Staff pose. Bend your knees, put your feet on the floor and slide your left foot under your right leg to the outside of your right hip.

Place the sole of your right foot on the floor just outside your left knee. Make sure that the right knee directly points up towards the ceiling.

Stretch your left arm up to lengthen through your spine and shoulder, then pass your left arm through the space between your chest and the right knee.

Reach your left arm along the outside of your right leg and take hold of your right foot or ankle so that your right knee is close to the left armpit.

Bring your right arm behind your back and place your right hand on the floor. Sit up as straight as possible. Keep your sitting bones down and your spine erect.

Inhale, lengthen your spine; exhale, twist to the right, moving your right arm, trunk and head simultaneously. Look over your right shoulder.

Breathe deeply and slowly. Use your left arm as a lever against the right leg to twist your trunk as far as possible without using the back muscles.

With each inhalation, elongate your spine; with each exhalation, twist a little bit more. If possible, you can also place the back of your right hand on the left side of your waist.

Stay in this pose for 20 to 30 seconds. Then return to the starting position, and repeat on the other side for the same length of time.

◆ The cause of bandha and moksha (bondage and liberation) is our own minds. If we think we are bound, we are bound. If we think we are liberated, we are liberated.

步骤说明

手杖式坐立。屈膝，双脚落地。左脚从右腿下方滑动穿过，来到右臀外侧。

右脚脚掌刚好放在左膝外侧的地板上。确保右膝向上直指天花板。

向上伸展左臂来拉长脊柱和肩膀，然后左臂穿过胸部和右膝之间的空间。

左臂沿右腿外侧伸出，抓住右脚或脚踝，使右膝靠近左腋窝。

右臂来到背后，右手置于地板上。尽可能坐直。保持坐骨向下，脊柱挺直。

吸气，拉长脊柱；呼气，向右扭转，你的右臂、躯干和头部同时转动。从右肩上方看过去。

深长而缓慢地呼吸。使用左臂抵在右腿上当作杠杆，不使用背部肌肉，尽量扭转躯干。

随着每次吸气，拉长脊柱；随着每次呼气，扭转再多一点。如果可以的话，你也可以将右手背贴放在左侧腰间。

在这个体式中停留20到30秒。然后回到起始姿势，换另一侧重复练习，停留同样长的时间。

◆束缚（bandha）与解脱（moksha）的原因在于我们自己的想法。如果我们认为我们被束缚住了，我们就被束缚了。如果我们认为我们无拘无束，我们就无所拘束。

Benefits

Half Lord-of-the-fish pose can help

· improve flexibility of the spine

· stretch the back and abdominal muscles

· massage the abdominal organs, promoting digestion and alleviating constipation

· relieve menstrual disorders, fatigue, lumbago and backache

Contraindications and Cautions

Women should avoid this practice during menstruation and pregnancy. People suffering from sciatica or slipped disc should not practise this pose. People with back or spine injury can only practise this pose under the supervision of a competent teacher.

Words and Expressions / 词汇表达

half [hɑːf] *adj.* 一半的   *e.g.* half month 半个月

lord [lɔːd] *n.* 主人，统治者   *e.g.* The Lord of the Rings 《指环王》

fish [fɪʃ] *n.* 鱼   *e.g.* fried fish 煎鱼

just [dʒʌst] *adv.* 刚好，恰好   *e.g.* just in time 及时，恰好

pass [pɑːs] *v.* 通过，经过   *e.g.* pass through 穿过

through [θruː] *prep.* 穿过   *e.g.* go through that door 穿过那扇门

take hold of 握住，抓住

erect [ɪ'rekt] *adj.* 直立的，笔直的   *e.g.* erect posture 直立的姿势

◆ It is only when we transcend the mind that we are free from all these troubles.

益处

半鱼王式能够帮助

· 提升脊柱灵活性

· 拉伸背部及腹部肌肉

· 按摩腹部器官，促进消化并缓解便秘

· 缓解月经紊乱、疲劳、腰痛和背痛

禁忌和注意事项

女性在经期和孕期应避免这个练习。患有坐骨神经痛或椎间盘突出的人不应该练习这个体式。背部或脊柱损伤的人只有在有能力的老师的监督指导下才能练习这个体式。

twist [twɪst] *v.* 扭转，转动（身体部位） *e.g.* twist off 拧开

look over 从……上面看

lever ['liːvə] *n.* 杠杆 *e.g.* lever rule 杠杆定律

without [wɪˈðaʊt] *prep.* 没有，不带 *e.g.* without a break 不间断地，不休息地

a little bit more 再多一点

if possible 如果可能的话，如有可能

starting position 起始姿势，开始位置

◆ 只有当我们超越了心意，我们才能从所有这些烦恼中解脱出来。

2.5.4 Paripūrṇa Nāvāsana / Complete Boat pose

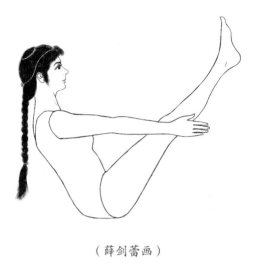

（薛剑蕾画）

Step-by-step Instructions

Sit in Staff pose and keep both legs extended. Place your palms on the floor a little behind your buttocks, fingers pointing forward.

With an exhalation, lean your trunk slightly backward and raise your legs off the floor, so that your thighs are angled about 60 degrees relative to the floor.

Balance your whole body on your buttocks. Straighten your knees and have your feet higher than your head.

Press less strongly with your hands, and finally extend your arms forward at shoulder level. See that your arms are parallel to the floor, with palms facing each other.

◆ Physical and mental toxins create stiffness and tension. Anything that makes us stiff can also break us. Only if we are supple will we never break.

2.5.4 完全船式

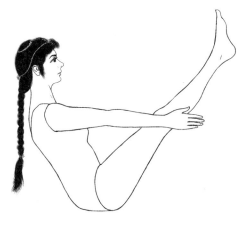

（薛剑蕾画）

步骤说明

手杖式坐立，保持双腿伸展。手掌置于臀部后面一点的地板上，手指指向前方。

随着呼气，身体稍向后仰，双腿抬离地板，让大腿与地板约成60度角。

整个身体平衡于臀部上。伸直双膝，让你的双脚高于头部。

双手下压力度减少，最后将手臂向前伸展与肩平齐。确保你的手臂与地面平行，掌心相对。

◆身心的毒素会制造僵硬和紧张。任何使我们僵硬的东西也可能将我们击垮。只有我们柔软，才永远不会垮掉。

Lift your pubis toward your navel, keep your spine firm and don't cave in your chest.

Gaze forward and stay in this pose for 20 to 30 seconds with normal breathing, imagining your body is floating weightlessly like a boat.

Exhale, lower your legs and hands back to Staff pose.

Benefits

Complete Boat pose can help

· strengthen the spine, abdomen, and hip flexors

· alleviate flatulence and gastric complaints

· massage abdominal organs, improve digestion, and reduce fat

Contraindications and Cautions

Women should not practise this pose during menstruation and pregnancy. This pose should be avoided in people with low blood pressure, diarrhea or gastrointestinal ulcer.

Words and Expressions / 词汇表达

complete [kəm'pliːt] *adj.* 完整的，完全的　　*e.g.* complete works 全集

boat [bəʊt] *n.* 船　　*e.g.* a small boat 一条小船

lean [liːn] *v.* 倾斜身体，前俯（或后仰）　　*e.g.* lean back 后仰，向后靠

angle ['æŋgl] *v.* 斜移，使成角度转向（或倾斜）　　*e.g.* angle the camera towards... 把相机对准······

◆ The essence of everything is the same, but it appears in many forms and names.

耻骨上提向肚脐，保持脊柱有力，不要含胸。

注视前方，保持正常呼吸，在这个体式中停留20到30秒，想象你的身体像一艘船轻盈地漂浮着。

呼气，放下双腿和双手，回到手杖式。

益处

完全船式能够帮助

· 强健脊柱、腹部和髋部屈肌

· 缓解肠胃胀气及胃部不适

· 按摩腹部器官，促进消化，减少脂肪

禁忌和注意事项

女性不要在经期和孕期练习这个体式。有低血压、腹泻或消化道溃疡的人应当避免练习该体式。

---

relative to 相对于

have [hæv] *v.* 使处于（某状态）　*e.g.* have the window open 让窗户开着

less [les] *adv.* 更少地　*e.g.* less fortunate 不太幸运

strongly ['strɒŋli] *adv.* 强有力地　*e.g.* blow strongly （风）刮得很大

finally ['faɪnəli] *adv.* 最终，最后　*e.g.* finally be solved 最终得到解决

◆一切事物的本质都是相同的，只不过以多种形式和名称出现。

pubis ['pju:bɪs] *n.* 耻骨

cave in 塌陷，凹进

gaze [geɪz] *v.* 凝视，注视　*e.g.* gaze out 向外注视，眺望

imagine [ɪ'mædʒɪn] *v.* 想象　*e.g.* just imagine 想象一下

float [fləʊt] *v.* 漂浮，飘动　*e.g.* float on 漂浮在……上

2.5.5　Setubandhāsana / Bridge pose

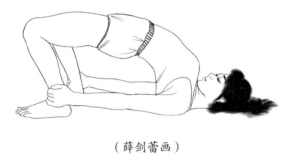

（薛剑蕾画）

Step-by-step Instructions

Lie on your back with both knees bent and your feet flat on the floor. Rest your arms alongside your body, palms down.

Move your heels close to the buttocks. Your feet and knees are hip-width apart.

Inhale deeply, pressing your feet into the floor, lift your buttocks upward and your chest towards the chin.

Raise your chest and navel as high as possible without straining

◆ If we could remember that basic Truth, we would never face disappointment nor get upset over the changes in the forms and names.

weightlessly ['weɪtləsli] *adv.* 无重量地　*e.g.* float weightlessly around
轻盈地飘来飘去
like [laɪk] *prep.* 像　*e.g.* look like 看上去像
gastric complaints 胃部不适

2.5.5　桥式

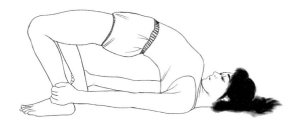

（薛剑蕾画）

步骤说明

仰卧，屈膝，双脚平放在地板上。手臂放于身体两侧，掌心向下。

脚跟靠近臀部。双脚和双膝打开与髋同宽。

深长地吸气，双脚下压地板，臀部向上抬起，胸部提向下巴。

保持双脚平放在地板上，大腿及双脚内侧平行的同时尽量抬

◆如果我们能记住这个基本的真理，我们就不会因为形式和名称的变化而感到失望或沮丧。

while keeping your feet flat on the floor and thighs and inner feet parallel.

You could bend your elbows and support yourself with hands underneath your lower back, or try to grasp the ankles with your hands.

To deepen the pose, clasp your hands below your pelvis and extend through the arms to help you stay on the tops of your shoulders.

Check that the body is supported by your head, neck, shoulders, arms and feet.

Hold this pose for as long as is comfortable. To come out of the pose, slowly lower down your spine vertebra by vertebra on the floor with an exhalation.

Benefits

Bridge pose can help

- keep the spine flexible and healthy
- strengthen thigh muscles and abdominal muscles
- stimulate abdominal organs and improve digestion
- reduce backache, headache, anxiety, fatigue and insomnia

Contraindications and Cautions

Don't practise this pose if you are in an advanced stage of pregnancy or if you have herniated cervical disc or advanced arthritis. People with neck injury can only practise this pose under the supervision of a competent teacher.

◆ Knowledge is a thing to be obtained from within by tuning in.

高你的胸部和肚脐，但不要勉强。

你可以屈肘，双手放于下背部进行支撑，或试着用双手抓握脚踝。

要加深体式，双手在骨盆下方紧扣，通过手臂伸展帮助你停留在肩膀顶端。

确保身体由头部、颈部、肩膀、手臂和双脚支撑。

在舒适的状态下保持这个体式。退出体式时，随着呼气，慢慢地让脊柱一节一节落到地板上。

益处

桥式能够帮助

- 保持脊柱灵活健康
- 强健大腿与腹部肌肉
- 刺激腹部器官，促进消化
- 减轻背痛、头痛、焦虑、疲惫及失眠

禁忌和注意事项

如果处于妊娠晚期，或者有颈椎间盘突出或晚期关节炎，不要练习这个体式。颈部受伤的人只有在有能力的老师的监督指导下才能练习这个体式。

◆知识是一种通过观照而从内在获得的东西。

Words and Expressions / 词汇表达

bridge [brɪdʒ] *n.* 桥   *e.g.* a small bridge 一座小桥

strain [streɪn] *v.* 使劲，竭力   *e.g.* strain for 竭力得到

2.5.6   Uṣṭrāsana / Camel pose

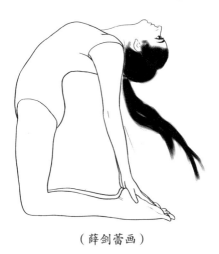

（薛剑蕾画）

Step-by-step Instructions

Kneel on the floor with your knees and feet hip-width apart. The tops of your feet should rest on the floor with the toes pointing back. Place your palms on the hips.

Inhale deeply, extend your thighs, lengthening and lifting your entire front trunk up. Tuck your tailbone in and roll your shoulders back to open your chest.

◆ "Tuning in" means to go in, to understand ourselves, to "know thyself" first. If we do not know ourselves, we will make mistakes in knowing other things.

> **grasp** [grɑːsp] *v.* 抓牢，握紧　　***e.g.*** grasp the yoga strap 抓住瑜伽伸展带
> **be supported by** 由……支撑

2.5.6　骆驼式

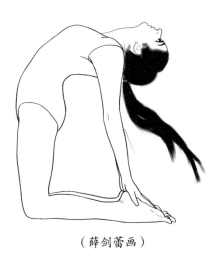

（薛剑蕾画）

步骤说明

跪立于地板上，双膝和双脚打开与髋同宽。脚背贴地，脚趾指向后方。手掌置于髋部。

深吸气，伸展大腿，拉长并上提整个躯干前侧。尾骨内收，肩膀后旋打开胸腔。

◆ "观照"意味着进入，理解我们自己，首先"了解你自己"。如果我们不了解自己，就会在了解其他事情时出错。

Exhale, keeping your chest well-lifted, curve your trunk back. Reach behind your body to place your palms on the soles of your feet. Point your fingers toward your toes.

Press your shins into the floor and your hands into the soles. Push upward with your heels into the palms as your pelvis arches forward and your cervical spine arches back. Use your hands to lift the chest further by moving your shoulder blades in.

Contract your buttocks and feel the stretch of your spine. Extend your head back.

Stay in this position for as long as is comfortable with normal breathing.

To come out of the pose, release your hands from your heels and rest them on your hips. Then sit on the floor and rest.

Benefits

Camel pose can help
- extend and tone the whole spine
- mobilize the shoulder and ankle joints
- correct drooping shoulders and hunchback
- relieve back pain and constipation
- reduce menstrual cramps

Contraindications and Cautions

People with high blood pressure, heart disease or lumbar disc herniation should not practise this pose.

◆ We must see if the mind is in a neutral position so it can judge things properly.

呼气，保持胸腔充分上提，躯干后弯。手来到体后，将手掌置于脚掌上。手指指向脚趾方向。

小腿胫骨下压地板，双手压向脚掌。在骨盆前拱，颈椎后仰的同时，脚跟推入手掌将身体向上推起。通过肩胛骨内收用双手进一步将胸腔上提。

臀部收紧并感受脊柱的伸展。头部舒展向后。

在舒适的状态下保持这个体式，保持正常呼吸。

退出体式时，双手从脚跟上拿开，放在髋部。然后坐在地板上，休息。

益处

骆驼式能够帮助

· 伸展并强健整根脊柱

· 活动肩膀和踝关节

· 矫正塌肩驼背

· 缓解背部疼痛及便秘

· 减少痛经

禁忌和注意事项

患有高血压、心脏病或腰椎间盘突出症的人不应练习这个体式。

◆我们必须看看思想是否处于中立位置，这样它才能恰当地判断事物。

Words and Expressions / 词汇表达

camel ['kæml] *n.* 骆驼

well [wel] *adv.* 很好地，充分地　*e.g.* well mixed 均匀混合

curve [kɜːv] *v.* 弯，使弯曲　*e.g.* curve the body sideways 侧向曲体

cervical spine 颈椎

2.6　Sūrya Namaskāra / Sun Salutation[⑩]

O lord and essence of light,

Lead me from the unreal to the real,

From darkness to light,

From death to immortality.

—*Brihadaranyaka Upanishad*

People in ancient times practised Sun Salutation on a daily basis as a way to worship the sun, Sūrya, because the sun has tremendous energy and is a powerful symbol of spiritual consciousness.

The best time to practise Sun Salutation is at sunrise or sunset. However, you may practise it at anytime that suits you the most as long as you practise on an empty stomach.

◆ The teachings can help you slightly, but too much learning may just muddle your mind. We should learn a little and work with that.

mobilize ['məʊbəlaɪz] *v.* 使可移动　*e.g.* mobilize the wrist joints 活动腕关节

drooping ['druːpɪŋ] *adj.* 下垂的　*e.g.* drooping eyelids 眼睑下垂

2.6　瑜伽拜日式⑩

主啊，光明的本质，

引领我从虚幻到真实，

从黑暗到光明，

从死亡到永生。

——《广林奥义书》

在古代，人们每天都要练习拜日式，作为崇拜太阳苏利耶（Sūrya）的一种方式，因为太阳拥有巨大的能量，是精神意识的强大象征。

练习拜日式的最佳时间是日出或日落时。然而，只要你空腹练习，便可以在任何最适合你的时间练习。

◆教导可以稍微帮助你，但是学习太多可能只会让你心意混乱。我们应该学点东西，然后运用起来。

Sun Salutation consists of twelve consecutive poses, which make the practice dynamic. Regular practice of Sun Salutation can bring health, energy and vigor into your life.

Step-by-step Instructions

Position 1: Pranāmāsana (Prayer pose)

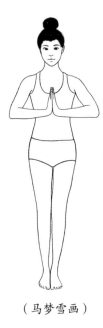

（马梦雪画）

Stand upright with your feet together or slightly apart.

Palms together in front of your chest.

Close your eyes and relax. Breathe naturally.

◆ Turning inside means turning the senses within; try to hear something within, see something within, smell something within.

拜日式由十二个连续的体式组成，使得练习充满活力。规律性地练习拜日式能给你的生活带来健康、能量和活力。

步骤说明

第1式：祈祷式

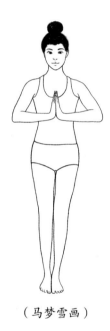

（马梦雪画）

站直，双脚并拢或稍微分开。

手掌合十于胸前。

闭上双眼，放松。自然地呼吸。

◆转向内在意味着让感官转向内；试着听到内在的声音，看到内在的东西，闻到内在的味道。

Position 2: Hasta Utthānāsana (Raised Arms pose)

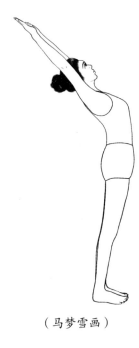

(马梦雪画)

Inhale, stretch your arms up above your head and gently bend back your arms, head and upper torso.

Keep your arms shoulder-width apart and the biceps close to your ears, palms facing upward.

◆ All the scents are within us. All the beautiful music is within us. All art is inside.

第2式：展臂式

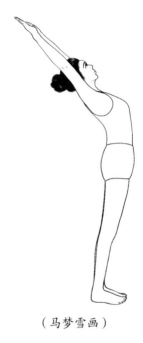

（马梦雪画）

吸气，双臂伸展向上举过头顶，手臂、头部和上半身轻柔地向后折弯。

保持双臂与肩同宽，肱二头肌靠近耳朵，掌心向上。

◆所有的气味都在我们心中。所有美妙的音乐都在我们心中。所有的艺术都在里面。

Position 3: Pādahastāsana (Hand-to-foot pose)

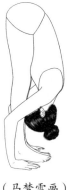

（马梦雪画）

Exhale, bend forward from the hips, and place your hands on the floor on either side of your feet. See that your hands and feet are in one straight line.

Try to bring your forehead close to your knees but without straining.

Keep your legs straight and your back flat.

Position 4: Āśhwa Sañchalanāsana (Equestrian pose)

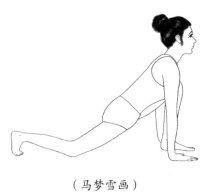

（马梦雪画）

◆ Many times people adore and worship symbols. Symbols should be used to transcend them. With the help of the mind, we transcend the mind. Once we reach our destination, we can throw it off and go away.

第3式：手至脚式

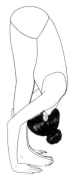

（马梦雪画）

呼气，从髋部开始向前折叠，双手置于双脚两边的地板上。确保双手和双脚在一条直线上。

尽量让你的额头靠近膝盖，但不要勉强。

保持双腿伸直，背部平直。

第4式：骑马式

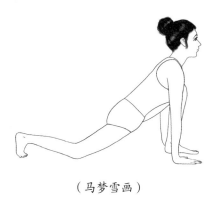

（马梦雪画）

◆很多时候人们敬慕崇拜符号。符号应该被用来超越它们。在头脑的帮助下，我们超越了头脑。一旦我们到达目的地，我们就可以扔掉它，然后离开。

Inhale, keeping both hands in place, bend your left knee and extend your right leg far back, with right knee on the floor and toes tucked under.

Release your buttocks down, move the chest forward, elongate your spine and look up.

Position 5: Parvatāsana (The Summit pose)

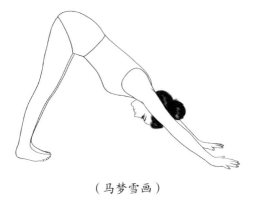

(马梦雪画)

Exhale, bring the right foot back beside the left foot. Raise your buttocks and straighten your arms and legs.

Flatten your back and lower your head between the arms. Try to lower your heels completely onto the floor.

Position 6: Aṣṭāṅga Namaskāra (Eight-limbed Salutation pose)

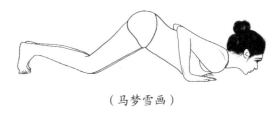

(马梦雪画)

◆ If the thought of hatred is in the mind, we can try to bring in the thought of love. If we can't do that, we can at least go to the people we love and, in their presence, forget the hatred.

吸气，双手位置不变，屈左膝，右腿伸展后撤，右膝落地，踮起脚趾。

臀部放松下沉，胸腔向前，拉长脊柱，向上看。

第5式：顶峰式

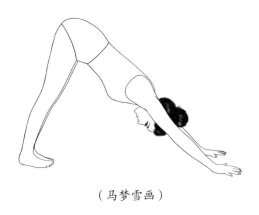

（马梦雪画）

呼气，右脚向后来到左脚旁边。臀部抬起，手臂与双腿伸直。

背部展平，头部垂于双臂之间。尽量将脚跟完全落到地板上。

第6式：八体投地式

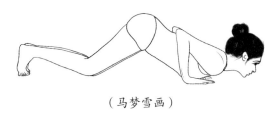

（马梦雪画）

◆如果心中有恨的念头，我们可以试着把爱的念头带进来。如果我们做不到这一点，我们至少可以走到我们所爱的人面前，忘记仇恨。

Keeping your breath held out, lower your knees, chest and chin onto the floor with hands beneath your shoulders.

Your buttocks, hips and abdomen are raised.

Position 7: Bhujaṅgāsana (Cobra pose)

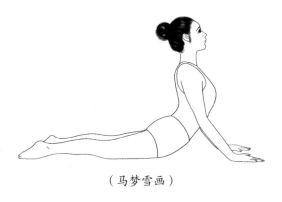

（马梦雪画）

Inhale, lower your buttocks while pushing your chest forward and up by pressing your palms into the floor.

Extend your legs and lower abdomen on the floor.

You can choose to straighten your arms or slightly bend your elbows, depending on the flexibility of your spine. Elongate the spine, arch back and look up.

◆ We can create a positive atmosphere by looking at a holy picture, by reading an inspiring book, by meeting with a special person, or simply by leaving the disturbing environment.

保持外屏息，双膝、胸部及下巴落到地板上，双手置于肩膀下方。

你的臀部、髋部和腹部向上抬高。

第7式：眼镜蛇式

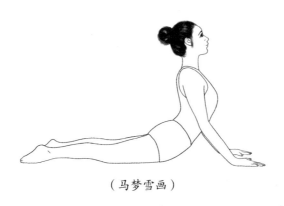

（马梦雪画）

吸气，手掌下压地板，推动胸部向前并向上，臀部下沉。

双腿及下腹部于地板上伸展。

根据自己脊柱的灵活度，你可以选择伸直手臂或微屈手肘。

拉长脊柱，挺胸后仰，向上看。

◆我们可以通过看一张神圣的图片，读一本鼓舞人心的书，见一个特别的人，或者仅仅是离开令人不安的环境，来创造一种积极的氛围。

Position 8: Parvatāsana (The summit pose)

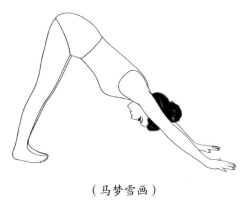

（马梦雪画）

Exhale, press your hands into the floor and raise your buttocks to come back to position 5.

Position 9: Āśhwa Sañchalanāsana (Equestrian pose)

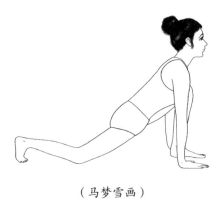

（马梦雪画）

Inhale, bring your left foot forward between your hands, with your

---

◆ Another way to control negative thoughts even before the thought overpowers us is to think of its after-effect.

第8式：顶峰式

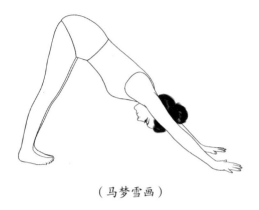

（马梦雪画）

呼气，双手下压地板，臀部抬起返回到第5式。

第9式：骑马式

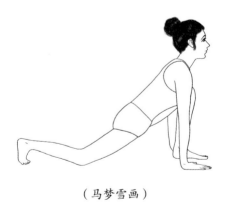

（马梦雪画）

吸气，左脚向前来到双手之间，右膝落地，踮起脚趾。

◆控制消极思想的另一个方法是在消极思想控制我们之前想想它的后果。

right knee on the floor and toes tucked under.

Release your buttocks down and push your chest forward.
Elongate the spine and look up to re-assume position 4.

Position 10: Pādahastāsana (Hand-to-foot pose)

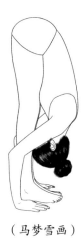

(马梦雪画)

Exhale, bring your right foot forward beside the left foot.

Straighten your knees and bend forward, bringing your forehead
towards your knees. Your hands remain on the floor beside your feet.

This is the same with position 3.

◆ With establishment in honesty, the state of fearlessness comes. One need not
be afraid of anybody and can always lead an open life.

臀部放松下沉，胸向前推。拉长脊柱，看向上方重新进入第4式。

第10式：手至脚式

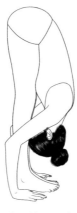

（马梦雪画）

呼气，右脚向前来到左脚旁。

双膝伸直，身体前屈，让你的额头靠向膝盖。双手保持放在双脚旁边的地板上。

这一步与第3式相同。

◆立足诚实，无所畏惧的状态便会到来。一个人不需要害怕任何人，可以一直过着开放的生活。

Position 11: Hasta Utthānāsana (Raised arms pose)

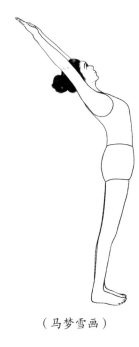

（马梦雪画）

Inhale, extend your arms up alongside your ears, raise your upper body and slightly bend backward.

This is a repetition of position 2.

◆ When there are no lies, the entire life becomes an open book. But this comes only with an absolutely honest mind.

第11式：展臂式

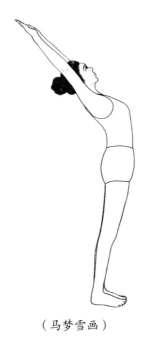

（马梦雪画）

吸气，双臂夹耳伸展向上，上半身向上抬起，轻微后仰。
这一步是对第2式的重复。

◆没有谎言，整个生活就变成了一本打开的书。但只有绝对诚实的头脑
才能实现这一点。

Position 12: Pranāmāsana (Prayer pose)

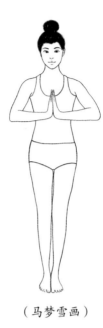

（马梦雪画）

Exhale, stand upright with palms together in front of your chest, and relax.

The above positions 1 to 12 complete half a round of Sun Salutation. In the second half, the positions are repeated with two small changes in Equestrian pose:

1. In position 16, extend your left leg instead of your right leg far back;

2. In position 21, bring your right foot forward between the hands.

◆ If by being honest we will cause trouble, difficulty or harm to anyone, we should keep quiet.

第12式：祈祷式

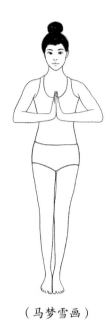

（马梦雪画）

呼气，站直，手掌合十于胸前，放松。

上面的1到12式构成了半轮瑜伽拜日式。在第二个半轮中，重复这些体式，在骑马式中有两处细微的调整：

1. 在第16式中，左腿而不是右腿伸展向后；

2. 在第21式中，右脚向前置于双手之间。

◆如果因为诚实会给任何人带来麻烦、困难或伤害，那我们应该保持沉默。

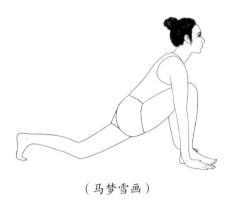

（马梦雪画）

This full round of Sun Salutation is performed for the sake of balance and can give equal stretch to each side of the body. Remember to lower your arms alongside your body, close your eyes and relax when you finish one cycle of 12 movements.

Benefits

Sun Salutation can help

· stretch, tone and loosen up all the muscles and joints

· massage internal organs of the body

· stimulate and balance respiratory system, circulatory system and all other systems of the body

· revitalize the body and mind

Contraindications and Cautions

Sun Salutation should be avoided in people with fever, acute inflammation or rashes. Do not practise this if you have high blood pressure, coronary artery diseases or have had a stroke. Women should

---

◆ Yoga is not a philosophy to be followed with blind faith.

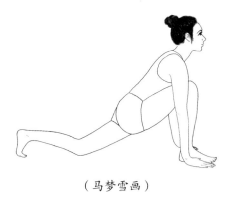

（马梦雪画）

做完整的一轮拜日式是为了达到平衡的目的并且能够均衡地拉伸身体的每一侧。当你完成一次12个动作的循环时，记得让手臂放下，垂于身体两侧，闭上眼睛，放松。

益处

拜日式能够帮助

· 拉伸、强健及松解所有的肌肉与关节

· 按摩身体内脏器官

· 刺激并平衡呼吸系统、循环系统及所有其他身体系统

· 恢复身心活力

禁忌和注意事项

有发烧、急性炎症或皮疹的人应避免练习拜日式。如果有高血压、冠心病或有过中风，不要做拜日式。女性不应该在经期和

◆瑜伽不是一种迷信盲从的哲学。

not practise Sun Salutation during menstruation and in the mid- and late-stages of pregnancy.

Words and Expressions / 词汇表达

sun [sʌn] *n.* 太阳　*e.g.* morning sun 朝阳

prayer [preə] *n.* 祈祷　*e.g.* morning prayer 晨祷

raised [reɪzd] *adj.* 抬高的，举起的　*e.g.* a raised teaching platform 抬高的讲台

equestrian [ɪ'kwestrɪən] *n.* 骑马，骑马者　*e.g.* equestrian skills 骑马术

far [fɑː] *adv.* 很远地　*e.g.* far away 遥远的

flatten ['flætn] *v.* 使变平，使平坦　*e.g.* flatten the yoga blanket 把瑜伽毯弄平

come back to 返回到

re-assume [riːə'sjuːm] *v.* 再采取　*e.g.* re-assume the old habit 重拾旧习惯

the same with 与……相同

repetition [ˌrepə'tɪʃn] *n.* 重复　*e.g.* repetition rate 重复率

above [ə'bʌv] *adj.* 前文述及的，上述的　*e.g.* above address 上述地址

a round of 一轮

half [hɑːf] *n.* 一半，半场，半程　*e.g.* cut in half 切成两半

small [smɔːl] *adj.* 不重要的，些微的　*e.g.* make a small mistake 犯一个小错误

◆ If we are true yogis for just one day, we will be transformed and want more of it. It's contagious, just like any other habit.

妊娠中后期练习拜日式。

change [tʃeɪndʒ] *n.* 改变，变化　 ***e.g.*** make changes 做出改变

full [fʊl] *adj.* 完全的，完整的　 ***e.g.*** full name 全称

for the sake of 为了

balance ['bæləns] *n.* 平衡，均衡　 ***e.g.*** ecological balance 生态平衡

equal ['iːkwəl] *adj.* 相同的，相等的　 ***e.g.*** be equal to 等于

remember to 记得

finish ['fɪnɪʃ] *v.* 结束，完成　 ***e.g.*** finish homework 做完家庭作业

loosen up 放松（肌肉）

balance ['bæləns] *v.* 使平衡　 ***e.g.*** balance work and life 平衡工作与生活

circulatory system 循环系统

revitalize [ˌriː'vaɪtəlaɪz] *v.* 使恢复生气　 ***e.g.*** revitalize dry hair 使干枯的头发焕发光彩

acute [ə'kjuːt] *adj.* 急性的　 ***e.g.*** acute diseases 急性病

mid-stage 中期

late-stage 晚期

◆哪怕我们只当一天真正的瑜伽士，我们也会有改变，并且想要更多。它（瑜伽）会传染，就像任何其他习惯一样。

Chapter Three
Yoga Nidrā

第三章　瑜伽休息术

> Most people sleep without resolving their tensions,
>
> This is termed nidrā.
>
> Nidrā means sleep, no matter what or why,
>
> But yoga nidrā means sleep after throwing off the burdens,
>
> It is of a blissful, higher quality altogether.
>
> —Swami Satyananda Saraswati

3.1 Definition and Importance

The word nidrā means deep sleep, and therefore, yoga nidrā is also called yogic sleep in some texts. Different from our daily sleep, this yogic sleep is a dynamic process accompanied by awareness. That is, one appears to be asleep in yoga nidrā, but the consciousness is actually functioning at a deeper level of the mind.

Yoga nidrā is a scientific method to help release and remove physical, emotional and mental stress. By practising yoga nidrā, one can achieve physiological balance and have better regulation of the mind and emotions. Meanwhile, yoga nidrā can help improve memory, productivity and focused attention. Moreover, one can not only achieve deep relaxation but also reconstruct and reform one's personality from within.

◆ All of us are thieves. Knowingly or unknowingly, we steal things from nature. With every minute, with each breath, we pick nature's pocket.

大多数人在没有解决紧张的情况下睡觉，

这被称为nidrā。

Nidrā的意思是睡眠，不管如何或为什么睡觉，

但瑜伽式睡眠的意思是卸下负担后的睡觉，

它全然具有极乐与更高的质量。

——斯瓦米·萨特亚南达·萨拉斯瓦提

3.1　定义及重要性

Nidrā一词意为深度睡眠，因此，在一些文本中，yoga nidrā也被称为瑜伽式睡眠。这种瑜伽式睡眠不同于我们日常的睡眠，它是一个伴随意识的动态过程。也就是说，在瑜伽休息术中，一个人看上去是在睡觉，但实际上意识正在头脑更深层运作。

瑜伽休息术是一种帮助释放并消除身体、情绪以及精神上的压力的科学方法。通过练习瑜伽休息术，练习者可以实现生理平衡并更好地调节头脑和情绪。同时，瑜伽休息术能够帮助提升记忆力、生产力及注意力。此外，练习者不仅能够获得深度放松，也能够重塑并改正一个人的内在品性。

◆我们都是小偷。有意或无意地，我们从大自然中窃取。每一分钟，每一次呼吸，我们都在扒窃大自然。

3.2 Hints and Cautions

1. Beginners should practise under the guidance of a qualified teacher and experienced practitioners can practise with the help of a recording.

2. Yoga nidrā should be practised in a quiet, private and well-ventilated room with appropriate temperature. Semi-darkness is suggested since people easily fall asleep in total darkness and find it hard to turn inward in bright light.

3. Avoid any physical contact with your neighbors if you practise with other people.

4. Dress in light and loose clothes. Cover the body, especially the feet, with a blanket since the body tends to cool down during yoga nidrā.

5. Yoga nidrā should be practised on an empty stomach. Please allow 3 or 4 hours for digestion after a heavy meal.

6. Lie down on a flat and comfortable surface, preferably your yoga mat. You are not advised to use your bed because the subconsciousness, in most cases, associates bed with sleep.

7. Try to remain alert throughout the yoga nidrā practice.

◆ We should receive each breath with reverence and use it to serve others; then we are not stealing.

3.2　提示与注意

1. 初学者应该在有资格的老师的指导下练习，有经验的习练者可以利用录音进行练习。

2. 应当在安静、私密、通风良好且温度适宜的房间练习瑜伽休息术。建议在半明半暗的环境里练习，因为在完全黑暗的状态下人们很容易睡着，而光线太明亮则很难转向内在。

3. 如果和他人一起练习，应避免与周边的人有肢体接触。

4. 衣着轻便、宽松。用毯子覆盖身体，尤其是双脚，因为在习练瑜伽休息术的过程中身体会冷却下来。

5. 建议空腹练习瑜伽休息术。请在饱食之后留出3或4个小时进行消化。

6. 仰卧于平整舒适的平面上，最好是你的瑜伽垫。不建议躺在床上，因为大多数情况下，潜意识会将床和睡眠联系在一起。

7. 尽量在整个瑜伽休息术练习过程中保持警觉。

◆我们应该怀着崇敬之心接受每一次呼吸，用它来服务他人；那样我们就不是窃取。

3.3　Yoga Nidrā: A Sample[①]

Step-by-step Instructions

Step 1: Prepare your body and mind

Lie on your back in Corpse pose, with your arms slightly away from the body and palms facing upward.

Keep your legs hip-width apart and your feet out to the sides.

Adjust your body, position and clothes to make yourself completely comfortable. When you are ready, gently close your eyes.

Take a long, deep breath and as you breathe out, you feel that all the worries of the day are gone.

Please keep your body still and stay awake during the practice. Mentally repeat "I will not fall asleep. I will keep myself awake throughout the practice" three times to yourself.

Feel that your breath is becoming longer and deeper and you become calm and steady.

Step 2: Make your own resolve

Now, it's time to make your resolve. Try to find your own resolve and express it in a short, positive and clear statement. Remember to affirm it in the present tense as an existing reality. When you are doing so, what you desire would be like a seed already deeply rooted in your mind.

◆ If we are completely free from stealing and greed, contented with what we have, and if we keep a serene mind, all wealth comes to us.

3.3 瑜伽休息术示例[①]

步骤说明

第一步：身心准备

挺尸式仰卧，手臂稍微离开身体，掌心向上。

双腿分开与髋同宽，双脚外展。

调整你的身体、位置和衣服，让自己感觉完全舒适。当你准备好了，轻柔地闭合双眼。

深长地吸一口气，随着呼气，感觉一天中所有的担忧都消散了。

请在练习过程中保持身体不动，保持清醒。在心里对自己重复三遍"我不会睡着。我会在整个练习过程中保持清醒"。

感受你的呼吸变得越来越长、越来越深，你变得平静而安稳。

第二步：下定决心

现在，是下定决心的时候了。设法找到自己的决心，用简短、积极、清晰的表述将它表达出来。记住，用现在时态，肯定它是业已存在的事实。当你这样做的时候，你想要的就会像是一颗种子，深深扎根在你的头脑中了。

◆如果我们完全摆脱了偷窃和贪婪，满足于我们所拥有的，如果我们保持平静的心态，所有的财富都会来到我们身边。

Step 3: Scan your body parts consciously

Now I will say the name of each body part. Please follow my instructions and mentally repeat the name you hear, be aware of it and relax it completely.

We will start from the right hand thumb. Index finger, middle finger, ring finger, little finger, palm of the hand, back of the hand, wrist, forearm, elbow, upper arm, shoulder, armpit, right waist, right hip, right thigh, right knee, shin, calf muscle, right ankle, heel, sole of the right foot, top of the foot, right big toe, second toe, third toe, fourth toe, fifth toe...

Now focus on the left hand thumb, index finger, middle finger, ring finger, little finger, palm of the hand, back of the hand, wrist, forearm, elbow, upper arm, shoulder, armpit, left waist, left hip, left thigh, left knee, shin, calf muscle, left ankle, heel, sole of the left foot, top of the foot, left big toe, second toe, third toe, fourth toe, fifth toe...

Now, take your awareness to your right heel, left heel, right calf muscle, left calf muscle, back of right knee, back of left knee, back of right thigh, back of left thigh, right buttock, left buttock, right hip, left hip, the whole spine, right shoulder blade, left shoulder blade, back of the neck, back of the head...

Bring your attention to the top of the head, forehead, right temple, left temple, right eyebrow, left eyebrow, centre of the eyebrows, right eye sinking and relaxing into the socket, left eye sinking and relaxing into the socket, right ear, left ear, right cheek, left cheek, bridge of the nose, right nostril, left nostril, upper lip, lower lip, points where two lips touch, tongue, chin, jaw, throat, right collarbone, left collarbone,

---

◆ Richness has nothing to do with momentary wealth. The richest person is the one with a cool mind, free of tension and anxiety.

第三步：用意识扫描身体部位

现在，我会说到每个身体部位的名称，请跟随我的指令，心中默念你听到的那个部位，觉知它并彻底放松它。

我们会从右手大拇指开始。食指，中指，无名指，小指，掌心，掌背，手腕，小臂，手肘，大臂，肩膀，腋窝，右腰，右髋，右大腿，右膝，小腿胫骨，小腿肚（腓肠肌），右脚踝，脚跟，右脚掌，脚背，右脚大脚趾，第二根脚趾，第三根脚趾，第四根脚趾，第五根脚趾……

现在把注意力放到左手大拇指上，食指，中指，无名指，小指，掌心，掌背，手腕，小臂，手肘，大臂，肩膀，腋窝，左腰，左髋，左大腿，左膝，小腿胫骨，小腿肚（腓肠肌），左脚踝，脚跟，左脚掌，脚背，左脚大脚趾，第二根脚趾，第三根脚趾，第四根脚趾，第五根脚趾……

现在，将意识带到右脚跟，左脚跟，右腿小腿肚，左腿小腿肚，右膝后方，左膝后方，右大腿后侧，左大腿后侧，右臀，左臀，右髋，左髋，整根脊柱，右肩胛骨，左肩胛骨，颈部后侧，头部后侧……

将注意力带到头顶，前额，右太阳穴，左太阳穴，右边眉毛，左边眉毛，眉心，右眼放松下沉到眼窝，左眼放松下沉到眼窝，右耳，左耳，右侧脸颊，左侧脸颊，鼻梁，右鼻孔，左鼻孔，上唇，下唇，双唇结合点，舌头，下巴，下颌，喉咙，右侧

◆富有与短暂的财富无关。最富有的人必是头脑冷静，没有紧张和焦虑。

right chest, left chest, middle of the chest, navel, abdomen, pelvic region, groin, right thigh, left thigh, right knee, left knee, right toes, left toes...

The entire right leg from hip to toes, the entire left leg from hip to toes, the entire right arm from shoulder to fingers, the entire left arm from shoulder to fingers, the entire trunk and head... Feel that all different body parts come back together again. Visualize the whole body as a complete one.

Step 4: Be aware of your breath

Become aware of your breath. Silently observe the inhalations and exhalations. As you inhale, feel the air flow through both nostrils into your body; as you exhale, feel the air leave your body... Imagine the energy flow is pervading every corner of your body...

Continue your observation of the breath with total awareness, and try to breathe through alternate nostrils. Inhale through one nostril and exhale through the other. Count the breath backwards from 54 down to 0. Inhale left 54, exhale right 54; inhale right 53, exhale left 53... Continue with your own breathing rhythm.

Slowly stop counting and again breathe through both nostrils. Mentally tell yourself "I am not asleep; I am practising yoga nidrā".

Step 5: Arouse opposite feelings and sensations

Now evoke the feeling of sadness. Try to bring the heart-breaking moments back to life or try to create a scenario in which you feel devastated. Feel the sadness, extreme sadness.

Now, feel the happiness within. Your heart is full of happiness and joy. Imagine you have everything you want and you are the happiest

---

◆ Changing all these world situations is not in our hands. We are not going to stop all these things. But what is in our hands is the ability to find joy and peace right here and now.

锁骨，左侧锁骨，右侧胸腔，左侧胸腔，胸腔中部，肚脐，腹部，骨盆区域，腹股沟，右大腿，左大腿，右膝，左膝，右脚脚趾，左脚脚趾……

整条右腿从髋部到脚趾，整条左腿从髋部到脚趾，整条右臂从肩膀到手指，整条左臂从肩膀到手指，整个躯干和头部……感受所有不同的身体部位又重新组合到了一起。想象整个身体是一个完整的整体。

第四步：觉察你的呼吸

觉察你的呼吸。静静地观察吸气和呼气。随着吸气，感受气体流经鼻孔进入到你的身体；随着呼气，感受气体离开你的身体……想象这股能量流遍你身体的每一个角落……

带着全然的觉知继续观察你的呼吸，尝试用鼻孔交替进行呼吸。吸气时通过一个鼻孔，呼气时通过另一个鼻孔。倒数呼吸，从54数到0。左吸54，右呼54；右吸53，左呼53……以你自己的呼吸节奏进行。

慢慢停止计数，再一次通过两个鼻孔呼吸。在心里对自己说："我没有睡着；我正在练习瑜伽休息术"。

第五步：唤起对立情感及感觉

现在唤起悲伤的情感。设法重现心碎的时刻，或创设一个让你感到崩溃的情境。感受那种悲伤——极度的悲伤。

现在，感受内在的幸福。你的心中充满了幸福与喜悦。想

◆改变所有这些世界局势并不在我们的掌握之中。我们不会阻止所有这些事情。但掌握在我们手中的是在此时此地发现快乐与和平的能力。

person in the world. Take a few moments to feel that happiness and enjoy.

Try to experience the sensation of heaviness. You are now in Corpse pose, and your body is becoming heavier and heavier. You feel your body becomes so heavy that you are unable to move a single part of it. You are just lying there, totally motionless and clung tightly to the floor.

Now arouse the experience of lightness, no heaviness at all. You feel your body is becoming lighter and lighter... Your body becomes so light, so light, as if you are a white cloud of smoke floating lightly in the air. Try to feel this lightness of your physical body.

Step 6: Visualize images

Now I will mention a few items and you should quickly visualize them in your mind instead of concentrating on them.

A small stream... a small stream... a small stream... colorful pebbles... colorful pebbles... colorful pebbles... soft sand... soft sand... soft sand... a pink rose with pleasant fragrance... a pink rose with pleasant fragrance... a pink rose with pleasant fragrance... green grassland beneath your bare feet... green grassland beneath your bare feet... green grassland beneath your bare feet... two birds happily chirping on a branch... two birds happily chirping on a branch... two birds happily chirping on a branch... wind rustling through the leaves... wind rustling through the leaves... wind rustling through the leaves... butterflies dancing beautifully under the sun... butterflies dancing beautifully in the sun... butterflies dancing beautifully in the sun...

◆ If we have decided to be happy, nobody can make us unhappy.

象自己拥有了所有想要的东西，**想象**自己是这个世界上最幸福的
人。花些许片刻来感受这种幸福，享受这种幸福。

努力去体验沉重的感觉。现在你处于挺尸式，身体正变得越
来越重。你感受自己的身体变得如此沉重，沉重到你无法移动任
何一个身体部位。你只是躺在那里，一动也不动，紧紧地贴在地
板上。

现在唤起轻盈的体验，没有一丝沉重。你感到自己的身体变
得越来越轻……你的身体变得如此轻盈，如此轻盈，你就好像是
一团白色的烟雾，轻盈地飘浮在空中。试着去感受你肉体的轻盈。

第六步：画面观想

现在，我会提到几个物体，在头脑中快速想象出它们，而不
要专注在上面。

一条小溪……一条小溪……一条小溪……彩色鹅卵石……彩
色鹅卵石……彩色鹅卵石……松软的沙子……松软的沙子……松软
的沙子……一朵芳香怡人的粉色玫瑰……一朵芳香怡人的粉色玫
瑰……一朵芳香怡人的粉色玫瑰……赤脚站在绿色的草地上……
赤脚站在绿色的草地上……赤脚站在绿色的草地上……两只鸟在
树枝上愉快地啁啾……两只鸟在树枝上愉快地啁啾……两只鸟在
树枝上愉快地啁啾……风穿过树叶沙沙作响……风穿过树叶沙沙
作响……风穿过树叶沙沙作响……蝴蝶在太阳底下翩翩起舞……
蝴蝶在太阳底下翩翩起舞……蝴蝶在太阳底下翩翩起舞……

◆如果我们决心要快乐，没人能让我们不快乐。

It's getting dark... It's getting darker and darker...

The outline of a snow-capped mountain... the outline of a snow-capped mountain... the outline of a snow-capped mountain... dark blue sky... dark blue sky... dark blue sky... the cawing of crows breaking the silence of night... the cawing of crows breaking the silence of night... the cawing of crows breaking the silence of night... twinkling stars... twinkling stars... twinkling stars... a bright full moon... a bright full moon... a bright full moon...

Step 7: End the practice

Now it's time to repeat the resolve you made at the beginning of the practice. Mentally repeat your resolve three times with full awareness.

Become aware of your body and the external surroundings and know that the yoga nidrā is coming to an end.

Slowly wiggle your fingers and toes. Gently move your hands and feet. With the next inhalation, reach your arms overhead and straighten your arms and legs at the same time, giving your body a stretch. Roll to your right side and rest for a few breaths. When you feel ready, use your hands to slowly push up to a seated position and gently open your eyes.

Words and Expressions / 词汇表达

prepare [prɪ'peə] *v.* 准备 ***e.g.*** prepare yourself 自己做好准备

clothes [kləʊðz] *n.* 衣服 ***e.g.*** put on clothes 穿上衣服

◆ Anything might happen. We need not bother about the future. Nor should we worry about the past. It has already gone. To be happy this minute is in our hands.

天色变暗……天越来越黑了……

雪山的轮廓……雪山的轮廓……雪山的轮廓……深蓝的天空……深蓝的天空……深蓝的天空……乌鸦的啼叫打破了夜的寂静……乌鸦的啼叫打破了夜的寂静……乌鸦的啼叫打破了夜的寂静……一闪一闪的星星……一闪一闪的星星……一闪一闪的星星……一轮皎洁的满月……一轮皎洁的满月……一轮皎洁的满月……

第七步：结束练习

现在是时候重复练习开始时下定的决心了。带着全然的觉知在心里将你的决心重复三遍。

觉察你的身体及外在环境，你知道瑜伽休息术就要结束了。

慢慢地摆动你的手指和脚趾。轻轻地动动双手和双脚。随着下次吸气，手臂高举过头顶，双臂双腿同时伸直，伸展一下你的身体。转向右侧卧，停留几个呼吸。当你感到准备好了，双手支撑慢慢推起身来到坐立位，轻柔地睁开双眼。

make [meɪk] *v.* 使得，使变得　*e.g.* make it right 使它成为对的，弄正确

◆任何事情都有可能发生。我们无须操心将来，也无须担忧过往。它已经过去了。这一分钟的快乐掌握在我们手中。

ready ['redi] *adj.* 准备好　*e.g.* get ready for 为……做好准备

breathe out 呼气

worry ['wʌri] *n.* 担心，让人发愁的事（或人）　e.g. no worries 不用担心

gone [gɒn] *adj.* 离去的，不复存在的　*e.g.* gone forever 一去不返

stay awake 保持清醒

fall asleep 入睡，睡着

throughout [θruː'aʊt] *prep.* 自始至终，贯穿　*e.g.* throughout 2019 2019全年

become [bɪ'kʌm] *v.* 变得　*e.g.* become beautiful 变美

calm [kɑːm] *adj.* 冷静的，平静的　*e.g.* keep calm 保持冷静

resolve [rɪ'zɒlv] *n.* 决心，坚定的信念　*e.g.* unshakable resolve 不可动摇的决心

it's time to 是……的时候了

express [ɪk'spres] *v.* 表达　*e.g.* express oneself 表达自我

short [ʃɔːt] *adj.* 简短的　*e.g.* make a short speech 简短的演讲

positive ['pɒzətɪv] *adj.* 积极的　*e.g.* make positive changes 做出积极改变

clear [klɪə] *adj.* 清楚的，明白易懂的　*e.g.* crystal clear 十分清楚

statement ['steɪtmənt] *n.* 表述，表达　*e.g.* personal statement 个人陈述

affirm [ə'fɜːm] *v.* 肯定　*e.g.* affirm a commitment to 肯定了对……的承诺

present tense 现在时态

◆ We are not going to change the whole world, but we can change ourselves and feel free as birds.

existing [ɪɡ'zɪstɪŋ] *adj.* 存在的　*e.g.* existing problems 存在的问题

reality [rɪ'æləti] *n.* 现实，真实存在　*e.g.* become a reality 变为现实

desire [dɪ'zaɪə] *v.* 想要，渴望得到　*e.g.* desire health 想要健康

seed [siːd] *n.* 种子　*e.g.* sunflower seed 葵花籽

already [ɔːl'redi] *adv.* 已经　*e.g.* already finished 已经完成

(be) rooted in 植根于，深植于

scan [skæn] *v.* 扫描　*e.g.* scan luggage 扫描行李

consciously ['kɒnʃəsli] *adv.* 有意识地　*e.g.* lie consciously 有意识地撒谎

say [seɪ] *v.* 说　*e.g.* hard to say 很难说

name [neɪm] *n.* 名称，名字　*e.g.* brand name 商标，品牌名称

follow ['fɒləʊ] *v.* 跟随　*e.g.* follow blindly 盲从

be aware of 意识到，觉察到

start from 从……开始

sink [sɪŋk] *v.* 下沉　*e.g.* slowly sink 慢慢下沉

socket ['sɒkɪt] *n.* 窝，穴　*e.g.* eye socket 眼窝

jaw [dʒɔː] *n.* 下颌

middle ['mɪdl] *n.* 中间，中央　*e.g.* in the middle of 在……中间

from...to... 从……到……

different ['dɪfrənt] *adj.* 不同的　*e.g.* different colors 不同的颜色

come back 恢复原状

again [ə'ɡeɪn] *adv.* 再一次，又　*e.g.* again and again 一再，再三地

visualize ['vɪʒuəlaɪz] *v.* 想象，设想　*e.g.* visualize success 想象成功

◆我们不能改变整个世界，但我们可以改变自己，感觉像鸟儿一样自由。

silently ['saɪləntli] *adv.* 静静地，默默地　*e.g.* wait silently 静静等候

observe [əb'zɜːv] *v.* 观察　*e.g.* carefully observe 仔细观察

leave [liːv] *v.* 离开　*e.g.* be allowed to leave 准许离开

flow [fləʊ] *n.* 流，流动　*e.g.* water flow 水流

pervade [pə'veɪd] *v.* 遍及，弥漫　*e.g.* (be) pervaded with 充满着，弥漫着

observation [ˌɒbzə'veɪʃn] *n.* 观察　*e.g.* careful observation 仔细观察

alternate [ɔːl'tɜːnət] *adj.* 交替的　*e.g.* alternate current 交流电

count [kaʊnt] *v.* 数数　*e.g.* slowly count 慢慢地数

rhythm ['rɪðəm] *n.* 节奏　*e.g.* a sense of rhythm 节奏感

arouse [ə'raʊz] *v.* 唤醒，引起　*e.g.* arouse fear 引起恐惧

opposite ['ɒpəzɪt] *adj.* 相反的，对立的　*e.g.* opposite direction 相反的方向

feeling ['fiːlɪŋ] *n.* 感情　*e.g.* hurt one's feelings 伤害某人的感情

sensation [sen'seɪʃn] *n.* 感觉　*e.g.* burning sensation 灼热感

evoke [ɪ'vəʊk] *v.* 引起，唤起　*e.g.* evoke a memory 唤起记忆

bring back to life 使重生，使复活

heart-breaking ['hɑːtbreɪkɪŋ] *adj.* 令人心碎的　*e.g.* a heart-breaking story 一个令人心碎的故事

moment ['məʊmənt] *n.* 片刻，时刻　*e.g.* at this moment 此刻

scenario [sə'nɑːriəʊ] *n.* 情境，场景　*e.g.* scenario analysis 情境分析

devastated ['devəsteɪtɪd] *adj.* 极度悲痛的，极为不安的　*e.g.* feel devastated 感到崩溃

extreme [ɪk'striːm] *adj.* 极度的　*e.g.* extreme anger 极度愤怒

◆ Serenity is contagious. If we smile at someone, he or she will smile back. And a smile costs nothing.

happiness ['hæpɪnəs] *n.* 幸福，快乐   *e.g.* pursue happiness 追求幸福

within [wɪ'ðɪn] *adv.* 在内部，在里面   *e.g.* from within 从里面，从……的内部

be full of 充满

joy [dʒɔɪ] *n.* 快乐，欢喜   *e.g.* tears of joy 高兴的泪水

a few 一些，几个

want [wɒnt] *v.* 想要   *e.g.* want to do 想做……

take [teɪk] *v.* 花费，耗费（时间等）   *e.g.* it takes 10 minutes to... 做……要花费10分钟

in the world 在世界上

enjoy [ɪn'dʒɔɪ] *v.* 享受，享受……的乐趣   *e.g.* enjoy everyday 享受每一天

heaviness ['hevɪnəs] *n.* 沉重   *e.g.* a sense of heaviness 沉重感

so [səʊ] *adv.* 如此，这么   *e.g.* so beautiful 如此漂亮

heavy ['hevi] *adj.* 沉重的   *e.g.* a heavy schoolbag 一个很沉的书包

single ['sɪŋgl] *adj.* 一个的（用于强调）   *e.g.* every single day 每一天

totally ['təʊtəli] *adv.* 完全地   *e.g.* totally different 完全不同

motionless ['məʊʃnləs] *adj.* 一动不动   *e.g.* remain motionless 保持不动

lightness ['laɪtnəs] *n.* 轻盈   *e.g.* a sense of lightness 轻盈感

light [laɪt] *adj.* 轻的   *e.g.* light industry 轻工业

a cloud of 一团，一大片

white [waɪt] *adj.* 白色的   *e.g.* white clothes 白色衣服

smoke [sməʊk] *n.* 烟   *e.g.* smoke alarm 烟雾报警器

◆平静是会传染的。如果我们对某人微笑，他或她也会对我们笑。一个微笑不需要任何代价。

lightly ['laɪtli] *adv.* 轻轻地　　*e.g.* hit lightly 轻打

in the air 在空中

image ['ɪmɪdʒ] *n.* 影，（头脑里的）形象　　*e.g.* digital image 数字图像

mention ['menʃn] *v.* 提及，提到　　*e.g.* not to mention 更不必说，更别提

item ['aɪtəm] *n.* 一件商品（或物品）　　*e.g.* end item 成品，最终产品

quickly ['kwɪkli] *adv.* 迅速地，快速地　　*e.g.* as quickly as possible 尽快

in one's mind 在某人的头脑中

concentrate on 全神贯注于，集中精力于

stream [striːm] *n.* 溪流　　*e.g.* main stream 干流

colorful ['kʌləfl] *adj.* 富有色彩的，多彩的　　*e.g.* colorful flowers 五颜六色的花

pebble ['pebl] *n.* 鹅卵石　　*e.g.* a white pebble 一颗白色鹅卵石

soft [sɒft] *adj.* 软的，柔软的　　*e.g.* soft soil 软土

sand [sænd] *n.* 沙子　　*e.g.* a grain of sand 一粒沙子

pink [pɪŋk] *adj.* 粉红的　　*e.g.* pink bubbles 粉色泡泡

rose [rəʊz] *n.* 玫瑰花　　*e.g.* a red rose 一朵红玫瑰

pleasant ['pleznt] *adj.* 令人愉快的　　*e.g.* pleasant scent 宜人的香气

fragrance ['freɪɡrəns] *n.* 香味，芬芳　　*e.g.* sweet fragrance 甜香气味

green [ɡriːn] *adj.* 绿色的　　*e.g.* green belt 绿化带

grassland ['ɡrɑːslænd] *n.* 草原，草地　　*e.g.* an open grassland 一片开阔的草地

bare [beə] *adj.* 赤裸的　　*e.g.* bare feet 光脚

bird [bɜːd] *n.* 鸟　　*e.g.* a little bird 一只小鸟

◆ A carefree life is possible only with a well-controlled mind, one that is free of anxiety, one without personal desires or possessions.

happily ['hæpɪli] *adv.* 快乐地，愉快地 *e.g.* sing happily 愉快地歌唱

chirp [tʃɜːp] *v.* 虫鸣，鸟叫 *e.g.* chirp louder and louder 叫得越来越响

branch [brɑːntʃ] *n.* 树枝 *e.g.* a broken branch 一根断枝

wind [wɪnd] *n.* 风 *e.g.* wind speed 风速

rustle ['rʌsl] *v.* 发出沙沙声 *e.g.* rustle in the wind 在风中发出沙沙声

leaf [liːf] *n.* 叶子 *e.g.* lotus leaf 荷叶

butterfly ['bʌtəflaɪ] *n.* 蝴蝶 *e.g.* butterfly effect 蝴蝶效应

dance [dɑːns] *v.* 跳舞 *e.g.* dance to music 随着音乐跳舞

beautifully ['bjuːtɪfli] *adv.* 漂亮地 *e.g.* beautifully designed 设计精美

get [get] *v.* 变得 *e.g.* get angry 生气了

dark [dɑːk] *adj.* 黑暗的，深色的 *e.g.* dark cloud 乌云

outline ['aʊtlaɪn] *n.* 轮廓 *e.g.* the outline of ……的轮廓

snow-capped ['snəʊ,kæpt] *adj.* 山顶被雪覆盖的 *e.g.* snow-capped mountains 雪山

dark blue 深蓝色的 *e.g.* dark blue ink 深蓝色墨水

sky [skaɪ] *n.* 天空 *e.g.* in the sky 在空中

cawing [kɔːɪŋ] *n.* 鸦叫声，呱呱叫 *e.g.* birds cawing 鸟群啼叫

crow [krəʊ] *n.* 乌鸦 *e.g.* Crow pose 乌鸦式

break [breɪk] *v.* 打破（沉默），打断（连续性） *e.g.* break in 打断（谈话，活动）

silence ['saɪləns] *n.* 沉默，寂静 *e.g.* the sound of silence 寂静之声

night [naɪt] *n.* 夜晚 *e.g.* good night 晚安

twinkling ['twɪŋklɪŋ] *adj.* 闪烁的 *e.g.* twinkling lights 灯火闪烁

star [stɑː] *n.* 星星 *e.g.* a red star 一颗红星

◆只有心意控制良好，脱离焦虑，没有私欲私产的人才能过上无忧无虑的生活。

bright [braɪt] *adj.* 明亮的   *e.g.* bright sunshine 明媚的阳光

moon [muːn] *n.* 月亮   *e.g.* a new moon 一轮新月

end [end] *v.* 结束，终止   *e.g.* end in... 以……结束

at the beginning of 在……的开始

external [ɪk'stɜːnl] *adj.* 外部的   *e.g.* external world 外在世界

◆ Sex is not the only way to show love. If love is based only on physical contact, the mind will never be satisfied with just one person.

surroundings [sə'raʊndɪŋz] *n.* 环境　*e.g.* comfortable surroundings 舒适的环境

come to an end 结束

wiggle ['wɪgl] *v.* （使）扭动，摆动　*e.g.* wiggle your fingers 摆动你的手指

◆性不是表达爱的唯一方式。如果爱仅仅建立在身体接触的基础上，那么心永远不会只满足于一个人。

Chapter Four
Prāṇāyāma

第四章　瑜伽调息法

The way you breathe is the way you think.
The way you think is the way you breathe.

—Sadhguru

4.1 Definition and Importance

What is prāṇāyāma?

The word prāṇāyāma consists of two roots: prāṇa and āyāma. Prāṇa means vital energy force which functions in various ways for the preservation of the body and is closely associated with the mind. Āyāma means length, extension, expansion, stretching and control. Therefore, prāṇāyāma can be understood as the expansion of the range of vital energy.

Once you start practising prāṇāyāma, you would soon realize that it is a series of techniques using the breath to control the flow of prāṇa within the body. Therefore, you may also say prāṇāyāma is the science of breath.

Why do we practise prāṇāyāma?

No one would deny that life exists no more if there is no breath. Breath is essential for sustaining all forms of life. By practising prāṇāyāma, the respiratory system and nervous system can be strengthened and purified. During the process of prāṇāyāma practice, more oxygen is taken into the body while toxins are eliminated and

---

◆ Teaching yoga is not like teaching history or geometry. The teacher must impart a life force — a little current — into others.

你呼吸的方式就是你思考的方式。

你思考的方式就是你呼吸的方式。

——萨古鲁

4.1 定义及重要性

什么是调息法（prāṇāyāma）？

Prāṇāyāma一词包含两个词根：prāṇa和āyāma。prāṇa意为生命之气，它以各种方式运作以维持生命，且与心智密切相关。āyāma意为长度、延伸、扩展、伸展及控制。因此，prāṇāyāma可被理解为生命之气范围的扩展。

一旦开始练习调息法，你很快就会意识到调息法是一系列利用呼吸去控制体内生命之气流动的技法。因此，你也可以说调息法是呼吸的科学。

我们为什么练习调息法？

没有人会否认，没有了呼吸，生命也就不复存在。呼吸是维持所有生命形式所必需的。通过练习调息法，呼吸系统和神经系统会得到强化和净化。在调息法练习的过程中，更多氧气进入体内，同时毒素被排出，压力得到释放。

◆教瑜伽不同于教历史或几何。老师必须把一种生命力——一股能量流——传授给别人。

stress is released.

Our breath is closely interrelated and interconnected with our body, emotions and mind. When the breath is calm, our body is calm, our emotions are calm, and our mind is calm. However, when our breath becomes agitated, our body, emotions and mind also become agitated. Therefore, we can say that breath plays such an important role in our life.

Although breathing usually happens unconsciously, we can still consciously regulate it. The main purpose of prāṇāyāma is to help us take control of the breath and ultimately of the mind.

4.2   Hints and Cautions

1. For the sake of safety, prāṇāyāma should be practised under the guidance of a qualified teacher.

2. Practise in a quiet, clean and well-ventilated place with appropriate temperature.

3. Prāṇāyāma should be done through the nose instead of the mouth. Make sure both nostrils are clean and clear.

4. If you happen to have a bad cold, skip prāṇāyāma and resume the practice when you recover.

5. Take a shower or at least wash your face, hands and feet before the practice.

6. The best time to practise prāṇāyāma is at dawn or just after sunset.

◆ However much make-up you wear, physical beauty will not last long. The real beauty is inside — in your character, your noble ideas, your aim in life.

我们的呼吸是与身体、情绪及心智密切关联的。当呼吸沉稳时，我们的身体是平静的，情绪是平稳的，头脑是冷静的。然而，当我们的呼吸变得急促时，我们的身体、情绪和头脑也变得焦躁不安。因此，可以说呼吸在我们的生活中扮演着至关重要的角色。

尽管呼吸通常是在无意识状态下发生的，但我们仍然可以有意识地调节它。调息法能帮助我们控制呼吸，最终控制心智。

4.2　提示与注意

1. 安全起见，调息法应当在有资质的老师的引导下进行练习。

2. 在安静、干净、通风良好且温度适宜的地方练习。

3. 调息法应当通过鼻子而非嘴巴进行练习。确保两个鼻孔清洁、通畅。

4. 如果你碰巧得了重感冒，那就不要进行调息练习，等身体康复后再继续练习。

5. 练习前沐浴或至少清洁面部、双手和双脚。

6. 练习调息法的最佳时间是在黎明或日落之后。

◆不管你化怎样的妆，外在美都不会持久。真正的美源自内在——在于你的品格，你高尚的思想，你的人生目标。

7. Regular practice at the same time and place is strongly advised.

8. Do not force your breath or practice beyond your capacity. Please remember practice is not competition.

9. Prāṇāyāma should be practised on an empty stomach. Wait at least 3 or 4 hours before the practice after meals.

10. Sit in a comfortable and meditative posture while practising prāṇāyāma. Keep your chest, neck and head in one straight line and your body relaxed. See that your body does not bend forward, lean backward or tilt laterally.

4.3   Abdominal Breathing

Step-by-step Instructions

1. Sit in a comfortable cross-legged position with your spine erect. Relax your shoulders and gently close your eyes.

2. Place one hand on your abdomen and the other one on your chest.

3. Inhale deeply and slowly through your nose while feeling the abdomen expand and rise.

4. Exhale through your nose and feel the abdomen contract to empty the air out of your body.

5. Feel your abdomen rise with each inhalation and fall with each exhalation. The hand on the chest remains almost still.

6. Do not force your breath. See that every breath is continuous

---

◆ Many times the gifts we get are merely an advance for a future obligation.

7. 强烈建议在同一时间、同一地点规律性地练习。

8. 不要强迫呼吸或进行超出你能力范围的练习。请记住，练习不是竞争。

9. 调息法应当空腹练习。餐后等待至少3或4个小时再练习。

10. 以舒适的冥想坐姿进行调息法练习。保持胸部、颈部、头部在一条直线上，身体放松。确保身体不前倾、后仰或侧斜。

4.3　腹式呼吸

步骤说明

1. 舒适地盘坐，脊柱挺直。双肩放松，轻柔地闭上双眼。

2. 一只手放在腹部，另一只手放于胸部。

3. 通过鼻子深长缓慢地吸气，同时感受腹部的扩张与隆起。

4. 通过鼻子呼气，感受腹部收缩，排空体内的气体。

5. 感受腹部随着每一次吸气隆起，随着每一次呼气下沉。放于胸部的手几乎保持不动。

6. 不要强迫呼吸。确保每一次呼吸连续、平顺。

◆很多时候，我们得到的礼物仅仅是对未来义务的预付款。

and smooth.

7. Try to practise at your own pace and maintain this steady breathing rhythm. After several rounds, end the practice with an exhalation and open your eyes.

Benefits

The abdominal breathing technique can help

· reduce stress and calm the mind

· cultivate awareness and improve concentration

· release tightness in the chest area

· prepare the body for more advanced prāṇāyāma practice

Hints and Cautions

Beginners are advised to attempt abdominal breathing by lying down on the mat or sitting in a chair maintaining a good posture. To check whether you are doing the practice properly, you may try to put a book on your abdomen and watch it rise and fall with each breath. Master this breathing technique before moving on to other prāṇāyāma exercises.

Words and Expressions / 词汇表达

abdominal breathing 腹式呼吸

cross-legged [ˌkrɒs 'legd] *adj.* 盘着腿的

empty ['empti] *v.* 倒空，使成为空的 *e.g.* empty the trash 倒垃圾

air [eə] *n.* 空气 *e.g.* air pollution 空气污染

fall [fɔːl] *v.* 落下 *e.g.* fall from... 从……落下

◆ A donation means something given just for the sake of giving, not for name, money or publicity.

7. 尽量以你自己的节奏来练习并保持这种稳定的呼吸节奏。几轮呼吸过后，以呼气结束练习，睁开眼睛。

益处

腹式呼吸法能够帮助

· 减轻压力，平静头脑

· 培养觉知，提高注意力

· 释放胸部区域的憋闷

· 让身体为更高级的调息法练习做好准备

提示与注意

建议初学者躺在垫子上或以良好的姿势坐在椅子上尝试腹式呼吸。你可以尝试将书放在腹部，观察它随着每次呼吸的起伏来检查自己是否练习到位。在进行其他调息法练习之前先掌握该呼吸技巧。

almost ['ɔ:lməʊst] *adv.* 几乎，差不多　*e.g.* almost done 几乎完成了

still [stɪl] *adj.* 静止的，不动的　*e.g.* keep still 保持不动

force [fɔ:s] *v.* 强迫，强加　*e.g.* force on 强加于，强迫接受

continuous [kən'tɪnjuəs] *adj.* 连续的，连绵不断的　*e.g.* continuous innovation 连续创新

◆捐款意味着仅仅为了给予而给予，而不是为了名声、金钱或宣传。

technique [tek'niːk] *n.* 技巧，方法　***e.g.*** new technique 新技术

cultivate ['kʌltɪveɪt] *v.* 培养　***e.g.*** cultivate talents 培养人才

be advised to（被）建议

attempt [ə'tempt] *v.* 试图，尝试　***e.g.*** attempt to do something 试图做某事

lie down 躺下

properly ['prɒpəli] *adv.* 恰当地，正确地　***e.g.*** behave properly 举止得当

4.4　Nāḍī Śodhana Prāṇāyāma

The word Nāḍī means the channel of energy and śodhana means purification. Therefore, Nāḍī śodhana prāṇāyāma can be loosely interpreted as the breathing technique that purifies or cleanses the energy channels.

Step-by-step Instructions

1. Take a comfortable seated position and relax.

2. Hold your right hand in front of your face and make a gentle fist. Extend your right thumb, ring finger and little finger, leaving the index and middle fingers tucked into the palm of your hand.[12]

3. First, close your right nostril with your thumb and inhale through your left nostril. Then, close your left nostril with your ring

◆ Accepting gifts binds us and makes us lose our neutrality.

watch [wɒtʃ] *v.* 观察，关注　*e.g.* watch something closely 密切关注某事

rise and fall 涨落，起落

master ['mɑːstə] *v.* 掌握，精通　*e.g.* master a foreign language 掌握一门外语

before [bɪ'fɔː] *prep.* 在……之前　*e.g.* before doing something 在做某事之前

4.4　经络清理调息法

Nāḍī这个词的意思是能量通道，śodhana则意为净化。因此，Nāḍī śodhana调息法可以大致解释为净化或清洁能量通道的呼吸技巧。

步骤说明

1. 选择一个舒适的坐姿并放松。

2. 右手放到面前，轻柔握拳。伸出右大拇指、无名指和小指，留食指和中指内扣于掌心。⑫

3. 首先，用大拇指关闭右鼻孔，通过左鼻孔吸气。然后，用

◆接受礼物束缚了我们，使我们失去了中立。

finger (and little finger) and exhale through your right nostril.

4. Continue your inhalation through the right nostril and then alternate to the left nostril to exhale. This is one round.

5. Remember, the pattern is: inhale, left; exhale, right; inhale, right; exhale, left. This prāṇāyāma, therefore, is also called alternate nostril breathing.

6. Please continue another 5 rounds with equal inhalation and exhalation, using the ratio 1:1. You may try to count numbers to help you measure the length of your breath. Increase the count as you are more experienced in this practice.

7. When you have fully mastered this technique, you can then increase the ratio from 1:1 to 1:2, which means the length of your exhalation is twice that of your inhalation.

Benefits

Nāḍī śodhana prāṇāyāma can help
  · nourish the body with abundant oxygen
  · calm and cleanse the nervous system
  · cultivate mental awareness and improve concentration
  · balance the left and right hemispheres of the brain
  · reduce stress and anxiety

Hints and Cautions

Practitioners should be familiar with abdominal breathing before embarking on Nāḍī śodhana practice. Be careful with the length of each breath. Take it slowly and the length of the breath will gradually increase without strain. Never rush to the result.

◆ We are trees growing in nature; all our energy, our actions, our thoughts, our words are the fruits of our lives.

无名指（和小指）关闭左鼻孔，通过右鼻孔呼气。

4. 继续通过右鼻孔吸气，然后交替左鼻孔呼气。这是一轮。

5. 记住，模式是这样的：左吸，右呼；右吸，左呼。这个调息法也因此被称为鼻孔交替呼吸法。

6. 请保持呼吸时间等长继续再做5轮，吸与呼的时长比例为1比1。你可以试着数数来帮助自己测量呼吸时间的长短。随着练习的精进，可以增加计数。

7. 当你已经完全掌握这一技巧后，可以将吸与呼的时长比例从1比1改为1比2。也就是说，呼气的时长是吸气时长的两倍。

益处

经络清理调息法可以帮助

· 用充足的氧气滋养身体

· 镇静和净化神经系统

· 培养头脑觉知并提高注意力

· 平衡左脑和右脑

· 减轻压力与焦虑

提示与注意

在开始练习经络清理调息法之前，习练者应当先熟悉腹式呼吸。注意每次呼吸的时长。慢慢来，呼吸的时长会没有压力地逐渐延长。不要急于求成。

◆我们是生长在大自然里的树木；我们所有的能量，我们的行动，我们的思想，我们的言语都是我们生活的果实。

People suffering from colds, fever or flu should not practise Nāḍī śodhana prāṇāyāma. The 1 : 2 ratio of inhalation and exhalation is not suitable for those with depression and heart problems.

Words and Expressions / 词汇表达

> **leave** [li:v] *v.* 留下　*e.g.* leave somebody doing something 留下某人继续做某事
>
> **pattern** ['pætn] *n.* 模式　*e.g.* consumption pattern 消费模式
>
> **ratio** ['reɪʃɪəʊ] *n.* 比例　*e.g.* sex ratio 性别比例
>
> **count numbers** 计数，数数
>
> **measure** ['meʒə] *v.* 测量　*e.g.* measure the width of 测量……的宽度
>
> **be experienced in** 在……方面有经验
>
> **mean** [mi:n] *v.* 意味着，意思是　*e.g.* what is meant by ... 何谓……，……的意思是什么
>
> **nourish** ['nʌrɪʃ] *v.* 滋养　*e.g.* nourish one's skin 滋养皮肤
>
> **abundant** [ə'bʌndənt] *adj.* 充裕的，丰富的　*e.g.* abundant resources 充足的资源

◆ "When the disciple is ready, the guru comes," is a well-known Hindu saying. When the receiver is well-tuned, the music comes.

有感冒、发热或流感的人群不要练习经络清理调息法。1比2
的吸—呼时长比例不适用于有抑郁症和心脏病的人群。

oxygen ['ɒksɪdʒən] *n.* 氧气　***e.g.*** oxygen bottle 氧气瓶

cleanse [klenz] *v.* 净化，使清洁　***e.g.*** cleanse the skin 清洁皮肤

hemisphere ['hemɪsfɪə] *n.* 半球　***e.g.*** northern hemisphere 北半球

practitioner [præk'tɪʃənə] *n.* 习艺者，习练者　***e.g.*** yoga practitioner
瑜伽练习者

be familiar with 熟悉

embark on 着手做

strain [streɪn] *n.* 压力　***e.g.*** under strain 处于压力之下

never ['nevə] *adv.* 从不，决不　***e.g.*** never quit 永不放弃

rush to 着急做，匆匆赶往

result [rɪ'zʌlt] *n.* 结果　***e.g.*** as a result 结果

be suitable for 适合

◆"当弟子准备好了，上师就来了"是一句众所周知的印度谚语。当接
收器调好后，音乐就有了。

Chapter Five
Yoga Dhyāna

第五章 瑜伽冥想

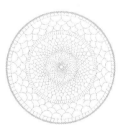

Be careful with what you meditate on. You want it —
you got it! As you train and then master the mind, gradually
the mind absorbs the qualities of the object of meditation.
Think of God[13] and you become divine.

—Swami Satchidananda

5.1 Definition and Importance

What is Dhyāna?

Dhyāna, or meditation, refers to a spontaneous state after deep
concentration in which the power of attention becomes so steadily fixed
upon the object of meditation that other thoughts do not enter the mind.
Therefore, meditation is a state of no-mind or, in other words, a state of
pure consciousness with no content. Each time the mind runs here and
there and you bring it back, that is called concentration. Concentration
is trying to fix the mind on one thing while meditation is when you
have tried and are successful.

Why do we meditate?

In this fast-developing technological society, we are faced
with changes, challenges and competition everyday. Pressure builds
up in our body and mind, causing so many physical, mental and
psychological problems. Meditation guides us to turn inward and
proves to be an effective way to counteract pessimism, depression and
tension. It can be utilized by everyone for mood control, to switch off

---

◆ All that is necessary is for us to tune ourselves. Then without even a
second's delay, the guru will come in some form.

> 谨慎选择你的冥想对象。你想什么——你就得到什么！随着你训练而后掌握头脑，而头脑也会逐渐吸收冥想对象的特质。念及上帝[13]，你亦神圣。
>
> ——斯瓦米·萨奇达南达

5.1 定义及重要性

什么是Dhyāna?

Dhyāna，或冥想，指的是深度专注后达到的一种自发状态。在这种状态下，注意力稳定地固定在冥想对象上，以至于其他念头无法进入到头脑中。因此，冥想是一种无念的状态，或者，换句话说，是一种无内容的纯粹的意识状态。每次思绪游离，然后你将它带回来，这叫作专注。专注是尝试将头脑固定到一个事物上，冥想则是你尝试了并成功做到了。

我们为什么要冥想呢?

在这个飞速发展的科技社会，我们每天都面临着变化、挑战和竞争。压力在我们的身体和头脑中累积，引发了诸多身体、精神及心理疾病。冥想引导我们转向内在，被证明是一种对抗悲观、抑郁及紧张的有效方式。人人都可以用冥想来控制情绪，关

◆我们所需要做的就是调整自己。然后上师会以某种形式出现，一秒都不会耽搁。

negative states and to replace them with states of well-being. Only when our inner being is in harmony, our interaction with the external environment can be harmonious.

5.2 Hints and Cautions

1. Beginners should practise meditation under the guidance of a qualified teacher.

2. Dress yourself in loose and comfortable clothes. Remove your shoes. Washing your face with cold water before practice can refresh your mind.

3. Find a clean, quiet and well-ventilated place to practise. Place a blanket or rug on the floor. Keep yourself warm with a blanket in cold weather. Keep insects and mosquitoes away from you and don't meditate under a fan in summertime.

4. Meditate in a comfortable cross-legged seated position, preferably padmāsana[14] (Full-lotus pose). Beginners may try to sit in sukhāsana[15](Easy pose) or ardha padmāsana[16](Half lotus pose).

5. If there is tension or stiffness in the body, practise several yoga asanas to relax. Only when the body is steady and still can deep meditation take place.

6. Keeping your mouth closed and breathing only through your nose can produce a calming effect. Close your eyes to avoid any visual distractions, which can also help you turn inward.

◆ When the heart is pure, you are always happy. Your concentration of the mind will come automatically without even trying.

闭消极状态转而用幸福状态加以替换。只有当我们的内在处于和谐状态时，我们与外界的互动才会是和谐的。

5.2 提示与注意

1. 初学者应当在有资质的老师的指导下练习冥想。

2. 衣着宽松、舒适。脱掉鞋子。练习前用冷水洗脸可让头脑清醒。

3. 找一个干净、安静且通风良好的地方练习。在地板上铺一块毯子或小地毯。寒冷天气下使用毯子保暖。远离蚊虫叮咬，夏天不要在风扇底下冥想。

4. 以舒适的盘腿坐姿进行冥想，最好是全莲花盘坐⑭。初学者可以尝试简易坐⑮或半莲花盘坐⑯。

5. 如果身体紧张或僵硬，练习几个瑜伽体式来放松一下。只有当身体处于稳定静止的状态时，深度冥想才会发生。

6. 保持嘴巴闭合，仅通过鼻子呼吸会产生镇静作用。闭上双眼避免任何视觉干扰，这样做也能够帮助你转向内在。

◆心灵纯洁的时候，你总是幸福的。你甚至无须努力，注意力会自动集中。

7. Meditation should not be practised after meal because the body is heavy and the mind is dull. Try to eat moderately, not heavily.

8. Regular practice at a fixed time and place is strongly advised. Start with perhaps half an hour's meditation daily and slowly increase the time.

9. It's best to practise meditation in the early morning and in the evening before going to bed. The best and the most congenial time for the practice of meditation is from 4 to 6 a.m., when the mind is calm and comparatively pure.

10. Don't fall asleep during meditation. To combat sleepiness, you could either go to bed earlier at night or take a shower before the practice, or both.

5.3 Guided Meditation: A Sample

Step-by-step Instructions

1. Sit in a comfortable cross-legged position with your spine erect to keep alert. Place your hands on the knees in Jñāna mudrā[①] (gesture of wisdom) or rest, one on the other, in your lap.

2. Close your eyes and relax. Take a few slow, deep breaths, with your entire mind watching the breath.

3. Then, slowly allow the breath to take its own course while continuing to observe it.

◆ Only an impure mind runs here and there, forcing us to bring it back again and again.

7. 餐后身体笨重头脑迟钝，不宜练习冥想。尽量适度饮食，不要过饱。

8. 强烈建议在固定的时间和地点进行规律性练习。起初每天冥想大概半小时，然后慢慢增加时长。

9. 最好在清晨或晚上睡前进行冥想。冥想的最佳和最适宜的时间在早上的4点到6点之间，这个时段头脑平静，比较纯净。

10. 冥想时不要睡着了。为了克服困倦，你可以晚上更早睡觉或者练习前冲澡，或两个方法都用上。

5.3　引导冥想示例

步骤说明

1. 舒适地盘坐，脊柱挺直以保持警觉。双手结智慧手印⑰置于双膝上，或上下重叠置于大腿间。

2. 闭上双眼，放松。做几个缓慢而深长的呼吸，头脑全然地观察呼吸。

3. 然后，慢慢地让呼吸自然发生，继续观察它。

◆只有不纯净的心智才会四处乱跑，迫使我们一次又一次地把它带回来。

4. After watching your breath, sit and quietly observe what is happening in your mind. Observe the thoughts and do not analyze or judge them.

5. You are just an objective witness. Whatever you see, you just watch and remain unaffected. These thoughts are just the different impressions previously recorded by your mind.

6. When your mind gets tired, you will find it settle down and rest in one place. Now, choose a mantra[18](for example, Om[19], a personal mantra given by your teacher, or any mantra based on your own faith), a word or any object of meditation that you personally like, and focus all your mental awareness on it. This calms the mind and makes it introverted.

7. Meditation begins with concentration and concentration culminates in meditation. It's natural that thoughts arise from time to time during meditation. If your mind wanders, just gently pull it back to the repetition of the mantra, the word or object of your focus. This is a natural process of meditation.

(silence for personal meditation practice)

Now focus on your breath again. Observe the flow of air in and out. When you feel ready, slowly open the eyes. May you remember the peaceful state of mind in the present and carry this peaceful feeling into your daily life. Oṃ śānti[20].

◆ We never lose by accepting pain. The more the pain, the more the gain— and no pain, no gain.

4. 观察呼吸后，坐在那里静静地注视头脑中正在发生的一切。观察这些念头，不要对它们进行分析或评判。

5. 你只是一个客观的目击者。不论你看到什么，你只是观察，不要受到任何影响。这些念头只不过是你的头脑先前记录下来的不同印记。

6. 当你的头脑疲惫了，它便会安定下来，停留在一处。现在，选择一个曼陀罗^⑱（例如，Oṃ^⑲，你的老师给你的私人曼陀罗，或任何基于你个人信仰的曼陀罗），一个词或任何你个人喜欢的冥想对象，并将你所有的头脑意识都集中在上面。这样做会使头脑平静、内敛。

7. 冥想始于专注，专注在冥想中达到顶点。在冥想时，时有念头升起是自然的。如果你的思绪游离，只需轻柔地将它拉回到曼陀罗念诵，拉回到那个词或你所关注的冥想对象上。这是冥想的自然过程。

（个人冥想练习保持安静）

现在再次关注你的呼吸。观察气流的进出。当你感觉准备好了，慢慢睁开双眼。希望你记得当下平和的心境并将这种平静的感觉带入你的日常生活中。Oṃ śānti^⑳.

◆我们永远不会因为接受痛苦而受损失。痛苦越多，收获越多——没有痛苦，就没有收获。

Words and Expressions / 词汇表达

guided ['gaɪdɪd] *adj.* 有指导的　*e.g.* a guided tour 有导游的游览

meditation [ˌmedɪ'teɪʃn] *n.* 冥想，静坐　*e.g.* meditation cushion 冥想垫

keep alert 保持警觉

wisdom ['wɪzdəm] *n.* 智慧　*e.g.* great wisdom 非凡的智慧，大智慧

lap [læp] *n.* （人坐着时的）大腿面　*e.g.* sit on one's lap 坐在某人腿上

take its course 任其自然发展

quietly ['kwaɪətli] *adv.* 安静地，静静地　*e.g.* sit quietly 静静地坐着

happen ['hæpən] *v.* 发生　*e.g.* happen to somebody （尤指不好的事）发生在某人身上

thought [θɔːt] *n.* 想法　*e.g.* at the thought of 一想起

analyze ['ænəlaɪz] *v.* 分析　*e.g.* analyze data 分析数据

judge [dʒʌdʒ] *v.* 评判，评价　*e.g.* judge by 根据……做出判断

objective [əb'dʒektɪv] *adj.* 客观的　*e.g.* objective condition 客观条件

witness ['wɪtnəs] *n.* 目击者　*e.g.* a witness to the car crash 车祸的目击者

unaffected [ˌʌnə'fektɪd] *adj.* 不受影响的　*e.g.* totally unaffected 完全未受影响

impression [ɪm'preʃn] *n.* 印记，印象　*e.g.* first impression 第一印象

previously ['priːvɪəsli] *adv.* 先前地　*e.g.* previously mentioned 先前提到的

record [rɪ'kɔːd] *v.* 记录，记载　*e.g.* record daily expense 记录日常开销

get tired 疲倦，累了

settle down 安定下来，平静下来

for example 例如

◆ Don't think that if someone causes us pain they hate us, but rather that they are helping us to purify ourselves. If we can think like this, we are real yogis.

personal ['pɜːsənl] *adj.* 个人的，私人的　*e.g.* personal information 个人信息

(be) given by 由……给予的

(be) based on 基于……

faith [feɪθ] *n.* 信仰，信念　*e.g.* religious faith 宗教信仰

object ['ɒbdʒekt] *n.* 物体，客体　*e.g.* object of study 研究对象

personally ['pɜːsənəli] *adv.* 本人地　*e.g.* personally speaking 就自己而言，就个人来说

like [laɪk] *v.* 喜欢　*e.g.* like doing something（平常）喜欢做某事

introverted ['ɪntrəvɜːtɪd] *adj.* 内向的　*e.g.* introverted personality 内向性格

begin with 以……开始，开始于……

culminate in 达到顶点，以……告终

arise [ə'raɪz] *v.* 出现，上升　*e.g.* arise from 由……产生，起因于

from time to time 有时，偶尔

wander ['wɒndə] *v.* 游荡，心不在焉　*e.g.* wander about 漫步，徘徊

in and out 进进出出

peaceful ['piːsfl] *adj.* 和平的，平静的　*e.g.* peaceful coexistence 和平共处

state of mind 心境，心理状态

in the present 在现在

carry...into... 把……带进……

daily life 日常生活

◆不要认为如果有人给我们带来痛苦，他们就恨我们，相反地，他们在帮助我们净化自己。如果我们能这样想，我们就是真正的瑜伽士。

Chapter Six
Communication Before
and After Class

第六章　课前及课后交流

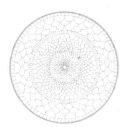

If you ask, you may get answers.

If you do not ask, there can never be an answer.

Asking is the way to learning.

—Swami Mantramurti

6.1   Communication Before Class

6.1.1   Greeting new customers

1. Namaste!②

2. Welcome to XXX Yoga Studio/Yoga Centre.

3. What can I do for you?②②

6.1.2   Catering for customers' needs

—I've never really done yoga before, so where should I start from?

—No worries. We have courses designed for beginners and the teacher will help you in class as well.

—Do you have any injuries, pain or health issues that you want us to know first?

—Yes, I once injured my ankle./ I have pain in my lower back./ I have high blood pressure.

◆ If flowery words make us happy but insults upset us, we know our minds are not yet strong.

如果你问，你或许会得到答案。

如果你不问，就永远不会有答案。

提问是学习之道。

——斯瓦米·曼特拉穆尔提

6.1　课前交流

6.1.1　欢迎新顾客

1. 向你鞠躬致敬！[21]

2. 欢迎来到XXX瑜伽馆/瑜伽中心。

3. 我可以为您做些什么？[22]

6.1.2　满足顾客需求

——我以前从没真正地练过瑜伽，应该从哪里开始呢？

——别担心。我们有为初学者设计的课程并且课堂上老师也会帮您的。

——您有没有受过伤，疼痛或者其他健康问题，想先让我们了解一下？

——是的，我脚踝曾受过伤。/我下背部疼痛。/我有高血压。

◆如果花言巧语让我们快乐，侮辱之词令我们不安，那我们就要知道我们的内心还不够坚定。

—Do you have any special requirements for today's practice?

—Well, I feel so tired after today's work and I hope to relax my neck and shoulders.

6.1.3 Yoga courses

—What kind of courses do you provide?

—We have a variety of courses written on this class schedule. Please allow me to introduce them to you. We have...

Aṣṭāṅga Vinyāsa Yoga

Flow Yoga [fləʊ]['jəʊɡə]

Haṭha Yoga ['haːtə]['jəʊɡə]

Integral Yoga ['ɪntɪɡrəl]['jəʊɡə]

Iyengar Yoga

Kids Yoga [kidz]['jəʊɡə]

Mindfulness Meditation ['maɪndflnəs][ˌmedɪ'teɪʃn]

Partner Yoga ['pɑːtnə]['jəʊɡə]

Prenatal Yoga [ˌpriː'neɪtl]['jəʊɡə]

Restorative Yoga [rɪ'stɒrətɪv]['jəʊɡə]

Yin Yoga

Yoga Therapy ['jəʊɡə]['θerəpɪ]

◆ A person who can only strike back physically may be physically strong but mentally weak.

——您对今天的练习有什么特殊要求吗？

——嗯，今天工作结束后我感到十分疲惫，希望可以放松一下脖子和肩膀。

6.1.3　瑜伽课程

——你们这里都提供什么课程呢？

——这张课程表上写着我们开设的各种课程。请允许我为您介绍一下，我们有……

阿斯汤加瑜伽

流瑜伽

哈达瑜伽

整合瑜伽

艾扬格瑜伽

儿童瑜伽

正念冥想

双人瑜伽

孕期瑜伽

复元瑜伽

阴瑜伽

瑜伽理疗

◆一个只能用身体回击的人可能身体强壮但心理脆弱。

6.1.4 Membership cards

—I am considering signing up for the courses here and try for a while to see how it goes, so what options do I have?

—We offer memberships for one month, one quarter and one year.

—Hmm...Maybe I will do one month. Just have a try first. If the courses here suit me, I will then renew my membership.

—Okay! That's a wise choice.

—What's the price of / How much is the monthly membership card?

—599 yuan.

—May I have a discount?

—Sorry, that's the lowest price we could offer.

6.1.5 Yoga props

—Do I need to bring my own yoga mat?

—You don't have to, but we encourage our customers to bring their own mat. Let me show you the props we have in the classroom. We have ...

blanket ['blæŋkɪt]

eye pillow [aɪ]['pɪləʊ]

folding chair ['fəʊldɪŋ][tʃeə]

hammock ['hæmək]

◆ When we have nothing to possess, we have nothing to worry about. All worry is due to attachments and clinging to possessions.

6.1.4　会员卡

——我想报这里的课程试一段时间看看，那我都有哪些选项呢?

——我们这里有月卡、季卡和年卡。

——嗯……我选月卡吧! 先试试。如果这里的课程适合我，到时我再续卡。

——好的! 您的选择很明智。

——月卡多少钱?

——599元。

——可以打个折吗?

——很抱歉，已经是最低价了。

6.1.5　瑜伽辅具

——我需要自带瑜伽垫吗?

——不是必须带，但我们鼓励顾客自带垫子。我带您看看教室里的辅具吧! 我们有……

毯子

眼枕

折叠椅

吊床

◆当我们没什么可拥有的时候，我们就没有什么可担心的了。所有的担心都来自对所有物的依恋和执着。

rope [rəʊp]

sandbag ['sændbæg]

yoga ball ['jəʊgə][bɔːl]

yoga block ['jəʊgə][blɒk]

yoga bolster ['jəʊgə]['bəʊlstə]

yoga mat ['jəʊgə][mæt]

yoga strap ['jəʊgə][stræp]

yoga wheel ['jəʊgə][wiːl]

6.1.6 Preparation before class

—What do I need to prepare before attending the class?

—Thank you for asking this question. There are several aspects I think every customer should pay attention to. Reserve a class one day in advance and if you can not make it, please cancel the class at least 2 hours before the class starts. Personally I strongly advise you to arrive 10 to 15 minutes prior to the class start time so that you have time to change clothes and talk to the teacher if you have any special requirements for the practice.

—Speaking of clothes, what do I need to wear and where do I change clothes?

—I would suggest you dress in loose and comfortable yoga clothes but please avoid those with a lot of exposure because we also have male customers here. You can change your clothes in our locker room and please remember to return the key to our front desk before you leave.

◆ Real samadhi means tranquility of mind, which is possible only when we dedicate everything and are free from all attachment.

墙绳

瑜伽沙袋

瑜伽球

瑜伽砖

瑜伽枕

瑜伽垫

瑜伽伸展带

瑜伽轮

6.1.6　课前准备

——来上课前我需要准备什么呢?

——感谢您提这个问题。我认为有几个方面每位顾客都应该注意。提前一天约课,如果来不了,请在开课前提前至少2小时取消课程。我个人强烈建议您在上课前10到15分钟到达,这样您有时间换衣服,并且如果您对练习有任何特殊要求可以和老师讲一下。

——说到衣服,我需要穿什么衣服?在哪里换衣服呢?

——我建议您穿宽松舒适的瑜伽服,但请避免穿太暴露的衣服,因为我们这里也有男会员。您可以到我们更衣室换衣服,走之前请记得把钥匙还回前台。

◆真正的三摩地意味着心灵的宁静,只有当我们奉献一切,从所有的依附中解脱出来,才有可能实现。

—Okay. May I have some snacks before class in case I feel hungry?

—Well, I would suggest you practise on an empty stomach. You might have some sweets or milk before you come here and you can use the bathroom right over there before class starts.

—Can I have my phone with me in the classroom? My boss or colleagues might contact me and I don't want to miss their calls or messages.

—Sorry. We request that all cellphones be turned off or silenced during class so that everyone can concentrate on the practice. I know you are busy but I guess you could call back when you finish the class.

—All right. Are there any other aspects I should pay attention to?

—Please remember to take off your shoes before entering the classroom and put back all the props after use.

—Sure, I will. Anything else?

—If you want to have some food or take a shower after your practice, please wait at least 1 hour.

—Thank you for your advice. I will keep that in mind.

6.2　Communication After Class

6.2.1　Asking for customers' feedback

—How are you feeling now? Do you still have pain in your lower

◆ Only a desireless mind, a mind free from everything, completely naked, can have peace.

——好的。万一课前我饿了，可以吃点零食吗？

——嗯，我建议您空腹练习。您可以来之前吃点糖果或喝点牛奶，课前可以用那边的洗手间。

——我可以带手机进教室吗？我的领导或同事可能联系我，我不想错过他们的电话或信息。

——很抱歉。我们要求上课期间所有的手机关机或静音，这样每个人都可以专注地练习。我知道您很忙，但我想您可以下课后再打回去。

——好的。还有其他我需要注意的方面吗？

——请记得进教室前脱掉鞋子，辅具用完后放到原位。

——当然，我会的。还有别的吗？

——如果您在练习完想吃东西或者洗澡的话，请等至少一小时后再做。

——谢谢您的建议，我会记住的。

6.2　课后交流

6.2.1　询问顾客反馈

——您现在感觉怎么样？下背部还疼吗？

◆只有无欲无求，从一切中解脱出来，完全放空的头脑，才能拥有平静。

back?

—Thank you. I feel much better after the practice.

—Do you have any suggestions for the course?

—I hope we could spare more time for Yoga Nidrā because it is so relaxing.

—What would you recommend to make the course better?

—The course is great! I personally expect the teacher to slow down the pace because I am a beginner. You see, sometimes it's hard for me to keep up the pace with others.

6.2.2 Offering suggestions

—I find it so hard to balance my body in the Tree pose and I notice that other people are doing great!

—Take it easy! I advise you not to push yourself so hard and don't compare with others in class. It's normal that you find it hard in the first few classes, but I can assure you the sense of balance will be improved with practice.

—I really want to try headstand! It looks so cool! Can you help me with that?

—Well, you'd better not attempt to do advanced poses before you master basic ones. I will guide you from the basics to the advanced poses, so please be patient and I am sure you will do headstand one day!

◆ Sometimes the mother feeds the child from a different plate just for variety, but the baby still eats the same food. It doesn't matter which plate we eat from as long as we eat.

——谢谢你。练完后我感觉好多了。

——您对课程有什么建议吗？

——我希望能留更多时间做瑜伽休息术，真的太让人放松了。

——为了让课程更好，您有什么建议？

——课程太棒了！我个人希望老师可以节奏慢一点，因为我是初学者。你知道，有时候我很难跟上别人的节奏。

6.2.2　给出建议

——我发现在树式中很难保持身体平衡，而且我发现别人做得太好了！

——放轻松！我建议您不要太强迫自己，课堂上不要和别人比较。最初几节课您觉得难是很正常的，但是我可以向您保证，平衡感会随着练习得到提升的。

——我好想试试头倒立！看上去太酷了！您可以帮我做一下吗？

——嗯，在掌握基础体式之前最好不要尝试高难动作。我会带领您从基础体式过渡到高级体式的，所以，请耐心一点，我确信终有一天您也可以做头倒立！

◆有时母亲用不同的盘子喂孩子只是为了多样化，但孩子吃到的还是同样的食物。只要我们吃，用哪个盘子吃并不重要。

6.2.3 After-class services

—Do you want some tea/water?

—Yes, please.

—We also have biscuits, sweets and nuts here. Help yourself!

—No, thank you so much. I am on a diet.

6.2.4 Saying goodbye to customers

—I'm glad that you enjoyed today's practice!

Hope to see you tomorrow!

—It's a pity that I can't make it tomorrow but I will come the day
after tomorrow!

—Great! Have a nice day!

—You, too! See you!

◆ Asana means the posture that brings comfort and steadiness. Any pose that
brings this comfort and steadiness is an asana.

6.2.3　课后服务

——您想喝点茶或白开水吗?

——好的。

——咱们这里还有饼干、糖果和坚果，自己随便拿!

——不了，非常感谢。我正在节食。

6.2.4　与顾客道别

——非常开心您享受今天的练习!

期待明天再见!

——很遗憾明天我来不了，但后天我一定会来!

——太棒了! 祝您过得愉快!

——你也是! 回见!

◆Asana（体式）指的是带来舒适和稳定的姿势。任何能带来这种舒适和稳定的姿势都是asana。

Appendix

附 录

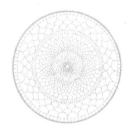

Appendix 1: Note
附录1：注释

① Aṣṭāṅga Yoga：音译为"阿斯汤加瑜伽"，意为"八肢瑜伽"，是胜王瑜伽的另一个名称。目前市面上开设的"阿斯汤加瑜伽"课程应为Aṣṭāṅga Vinyāsa，请读者注意区分。

② Nāḍī: channel of energy. It is said that there are 7200 nāḍīis, of which 3 are the most important. They are iḍā nāḍī (channel of lunar energy), piṅgalā nāḍī (channel of solar energy) and suṣumnā nāḍī (central energy channel).
纳迪：能量通道。据说有7200条能量通道，其中有3条最为重要，分别是左脉（阴性能量通道），右脉（阳性能量通道）和中脉（中间能量通道）。

③ Cakra: The word cakra literally means "wheel". It is the centre of energy or psychic centre. The seven cakras from bottom to up are root cakra (Mūlādhāra cakra), sacral cakra (Svādhiṣṭhāna cakra), navel cakra (Maṇipūra cakra), heart cakra (Anāhata cakra), throat cakra (Viśuddha cakra), third-eye cakra (Ājñā cakra) and and crown cakra (Sahasrāra cakra).

◆ A person who lives a minimalist lifestyle with the bare is free from bother.

脉轮：Cakra这个词的字面意思是"轮"。它是能量中心或精神中心。七个脉轮自下而上分别为根轮（Mūlādhāra cakra）、骶骨轮（Svādhiṣṭhāna cakra）、脐轮（Maṇipūra cakra）、心轮（Anāhata cakra）、喉轮（Viśuddha cakra）、眉心轮（Ājñā cakra）和顶轮（Sahasrāra cakra）。

④ 三角伸展式（Utthita Trikoṇāsana / Extended Triangle pose）：在三角伸展式及后续的战士一式中，教师应当根据会员身体情况灵活调整双脚之间打开的距离。目前越来越多英语国家人士使用公制（metric system），因此，英文口令将"米"（metre）放在口令正文部分，考虑到部分国家及地区的人仍习惯用英制（British system），特将"foot"（英尺）附在括号里，供读者在教学活动中根据教学对象按需选用。同样的问题和处理办法适用于2.1.5 章节的战士一式，敬请读者朋友们注意。

⑤ Makarāsana (Crocodile pose)：The instructions used in the text can be considered as instructions of Crocodile Rest pose (*The Yoga Toolbox*, 2010, p.54). Besides extending your legs hip-width apart and resting the tops of feet on the floor, you could also separate your legs slightly wider than your hips with the inner feet on the floor. Basically, this is a pose you can perform whenever you feel tired in yoga class. Also, you can use it as a transitional pose to help you get prepared for the next prone posture. The traditional way of performing Crocodile pose is to raise your head and shoulders with your elbows on the floor and your chin supported by your palms (*Asana Pranayama Mudra*

◆一个过着极简生活的人没有烦恼。

Bandha, 2013, p.111).

鳄鱼式：文中使用的口令可以看作是鳄鱼休息式的口令（《瑜伽工具箱》，2010，p.54）。除了双腿伸展与髋同宽，脚背贴地的做法之外，还可以双腿分开略比胯宽，双脚内侧着地。从根本上来说，这是一个在瑜伽课上你随时可以用来放松的体式。此外，你还可以将它用作进入下一个俯卧体式的过渡体式。鳄鱼式的传统做法是头部和肩膀抬起，手肘撑地，手掌托住下巴（《体位法 调息法 契合法 收束法》，2013，p.111）。

⑥ Śalabhāsana (Locust pose) : You could also try this pose with arms by the sides of your body (*Asana Pranayama Mudra Bandha*, 2013, p.249), with the palms facing the thighs (*Integral Yoga Hatha for Beginners*, 2009, p. 13), with the hands clenched (*Asana Pranayama Mudra Bandha*, 2013, p.249), or with your head and chest lifted and your arms stretched backward while raising both legs(《健身瑜伽体位标准（试行）》, 2018, p.80).

蝗虫式：你也可以通过以下方式尝试这个体式：双臂置于身体两侧（《体位法 调息法 契合法 收束法》，2013，p.249）；手掌朝向大腿（《适合初学者的整合瑜伽哈达》，2009，p.13）；双手紧握（《体位法 调息法 契合法 收束法》，2013，p.249）；或者抬起双腿的同时抬起你的头部、胸部，双臂后展（《健身瑜伽体位标准（试行）》，2018，p.80）。

⑦ Viparīta Karaṇī (Legs-up-the-wall pose) : Traditionally, this pose can be seen as a preparatory practice for shoulder stand. The traditional

---

◆ To have maximum and endless joy, learn to be non-attached. That doesn't mean ignoring people or having no feelings about them, but means avoiding selfish attachment.

way of performing this pose is supporting your body with hands, upper arms, shoulders and neck, with the trunk at a 45-degree angle to the floor and legs extended upward (*Asana Pranayama Mudra Bandha*, 2013, pp. 308-309). The version introduced here, which is frequently seen in yoga classes, is easier and safer to practise. Viparīta means "inverted", karaṇī means "doing, a particular type of practice". The most commonly seen English translation of this pose—"Legs-up-the-wall pose"—reveals how westerners usually perform this pose. However, Chinese people try to use imagination to describe the image of this pose and hence the name "inverted scissors" or "inverted arrow". When translating the name of this pose into Chinese, I also added the element/prop — the wall.

靠墙倒剪式：传统上，这个体式可以看作肩倒立的准备练习。这个体式的传统做法是用手、大臂、肩膀和脖子支撑身体，躯干与地面呈45度角，腿向上伸展（《体位法 调息法 契合法 收束法》，2013，pp.308—309）。这里介绍的这个版本在瑜伽课上很常见，练习起来更容易也更安全。Viparīta意为"倒置"，karaṇī意为"做，一种特定的实践"。这个体式最常见的英文译名——"腿上墙式"——揭示出西方人做这个体式的惯常做法。而中国人则试图用想象来描述这个体式的形象，因此有了"倒剪"或"倒箭"的名字。在将这个体式名称译为中文时，我也加入了墙这一元素/辅具。

⑧ Bandha: It means the postural contraction of the body, or the psycho-muscular energy locks which close the pranic exits (like throat,

---

◆要想获得无上无尽的快乐，就要学会不依附。这并不意味着要忽视别人或对他们没有感情，而是要避免自私的依附。

anus, etc) (see *Sanskrit Glossary of Yogic Terms*, 2007, p.35). There are four bandhas: Jālandhāra Bandha (throat lock), Mūla Bandha (perineum contraction), Uḍḍīyāna Bandha (abdominal contraction) and Mahā Bandha (the great lock), which is the combination of the first three bandhas (*Asana Pranayama Mudra Bandha*, 2013, pp. 545-558). In this context, the bandha particularly refers to abdominal contraction, and in real teaching you could say "gently engage the core".

能量锁（音译为"班达"，又译为"收束""锁印"）：身体的姿势性收缩；精神—肌肉能量锁，是关闭生命之气的出口（如喉咙、肛门等）（参见《瑜伽术语梵文词汇》，2007，p.35）。能量锁有四种：喉锁、根锁（会阴收束）、腹锁和大收束法，大收束法是前三种的结合（《体位法 调息法 契合法 收束法》，2013，pp.545—558）。在这个语境中，"bandha"特指腹部收缩。在实际教学中，可以说"轻柔地收紧核心"。

⑨ Mārjāriāsana: mārjāri意为"猫"，因此，在有的书籍中，该体式译为"猫伸展式"，涵盖两个动态动作。（*Asana Pranayama Mudra Bandha*, 2013, p.148）但在实际信息检索过程中发现有些书籍及流派将该体式拆分为两个体式，合称"猫牛式"（Cat-Cow pose），并且用Mārjāriāsana泛化指代两个体式（见*Yoga Toolbox for Teachers and Students*）。当然，也有将猫牛式拆开列为两个单独的体式（见https://www.yogajournal.com.au/pose-finder/），分别称"猫式"（Mārjāriāsana / Cat Pose）和"牛式"（Bītilāsana / Cow pose）。本书采用"猫伸展式"作为译名，在中英文口令中用括号注释了猫牛式的明确定位，即"吸气，背部下凹，牛式；

◆ The world has been created for us to understand, to make use of, and to grow in.

呼气，背部拱起，猫式"，便于读者在日常教学及学习中灵活使用。

⑩ Sūrya Namaskāra: This sequence is based on the book *Asana Pranayama Mudra Bandha* (2013) written by Swami Satyananda Saraswati. However, we should be aware that the sequence of Sūrya Namaskāra varies in different schools of yoga. Even when it comes to the traditional type, differences still exist.

瑜伽拜日式：本序列基于斯瓦米·萨特亚南达·萨拉斯瓦提所著《体位法 调息法 契合法 收束法》(2013) 一书。然而，我们应该意识到拜日式的序列因瑜伽流派不同而各异，甚至单说传统类型，差异也是存在的。

⑪ Yoga Nidrā: A Sample: The outline of this yoga nidrā sample is based on the book *Yoga Nidrā* (2013) written by Swami Satyananda Saraswati. *Yoga Nidrā* is one of the most classical books illustrating yoga nidrā with detailed yet clear explanations, procedures and examples.

瑜伽休息术示例：这个瑜伽休息术示例的大纲是基于斯瓦米·萨特亚南达·萨拉斯瓦提所写的《瑜伽休息术》（2013）一书。《瑜伽休息术》是阐述瑜伽休息术最为经典的书籍之一，它提供了详细而清晰的解释、步骤及范例。

⑫ Please note that the hand gesture used in prāṇāyāma may vary in different schools of yoga. Besides what I introduced in the text, you may also rest your index finger and middle finger on the centre of your eyebrows and use your thumb and ring finger to control the flow of breath in your right nostril and left nostril respectively. (*Asana Pranayama Mudra Bandha*, 2013, p.457)

请注意不同瑜伽流派中的调息手势可能会有所不同。除了我在文中介绍的方法，你也可以将食指和中指放在眉心处，用大拇指和无名指分别控制右鼻孔和左鼻孔的气息流动。（《体位法 调息法 契合法 收束法》，2013，p.457）

⑬ God: Please note that here the word "God" contains no religious meaning. In *The Yoga Sutras of Patanjali* (2008), Swami Satchidananda said, "What is God? Peace, contentment, egolessness. " (p.200) These are the qualities of eternal happiness. Moreover, in *To Know Your Self* (2008), Swami Satchidananda again explained the meaning of God by saying "You are happiness personified...You are the image of happiness. If you want to use the word God, who is God? What are God's qualifications? Always being happy...Nobody can always be completely happy without knowing that he or she is happiness. This is what God is. " (p.8, p.10)

上帝：请注意这里的"上帝"一词并无宗教意义。在《帕坦加利的瑜伽经》（2008）中，斯瓦米·萨奇达南达说："上帝是什么？是和平、满足和无我。"（p.200）这些都是永恒幸福的品质。此外，在《认识你的真我》（2008）中，斯瓦米·萨奇达南达再次解释了上帝的意义。他说："你是幸福的化身……你是幸福的形象。如果你想用上帝这个词，上帝是谁？上帝的资格是什

◆ A perfect action should not bring harm to anybody, including yourself.

么？永远幸福……如果不知道他/她自己就是幸福本身，没有人能永远完全幸福。这就是上帝。"（p.8，p.10）

⑭ Padmāsana (Full lotus pose): Sit with both legs bent and feet placed on the top of the opposite thighs. See that the soles of feet face upward and heels touch the pelvic bone.

全莲花坐：坐立，曲双腿，双脚置于对侧大腿上方。确保双脚脚心朝上，脚跟贴髋骨。

⑮ Sukhāsana (Easy pose): Sit with your right foot under the left thigh and your left foot under the right thigh.

简易坐：坐立，右脚置于左大腿下方，左脚置于右大腿下方。

⑯ Ardha Padmāsana (Half-lotus pose): Sit with one leg bent and the foot placed on the inside of the opposite thigh while the other leg bent and the foot placed on top of the opposite thigh.

半莲花坐：坐立，单腿屈腿，脚贴在对侧大腿内侧，曲另一条腿，脚置于对侧大腿上方。

⑰ Jñāna mudrā: Mudrā is a sealing posture, which refers to a movement or position made or taken by the fingers or limbs in meditation. Jñāna mudrā is a hand gesture in which the tip of the index finger is brought in contact with the tip of the thumb, while the remaining three fingers are kept extended. The gesture is a symbol of intuitive knowledge and wisdom (jñāna).

◆完美的行为不应该给任何人带来伤害，包括你自己。

智慧手印：Mudrā是一个封印姿势，指的是在冥想时用手指（称为手印）或肢体（称为身印）做出的动作。智慧手印是食指指尖与拇指指尖相触，其余三指伸展的手印。这一手印是直觉知识与智慧（jñāna）的象征。

⑱ Mantra: Mantra refers to subtle sound vibration. A mantra can be a syllable, a word or a sentence. The effect of chanting mantra lies not in its intellectual meaning but in its inherent sound-power.

曼陀罗：Mantra指的是精微的声音振动。一个曼陀罗可以是一个音节、一个词或一句话。曼陀罗唱诵的作用不在词意上而在于其内在的声音力量。

⑲ Om: In the tradition of yoga, Om (or AUM) is considered to be the primordial seed of the universe and, therefore, the supreme mantra. Om is not used for religious purpose in yoga practice. Rather, it is merely a means for practitioners to calm down.

Om：在瑜伽传统中，Om（或AUM）被视为宇宙的初始之音，因此也是至高无上的曼陀罗。在瑜伽练习中，Om并不用作宗教目的。确切地说，它只是一个帮助习练者平静下来的方法而已。

⑳ Om śānti: śānti means peace, pacification, and tranquility. Om śānti, the combination of two mantras, offers us a strong, positive vibration and an entirely new energy to work with. When we chant śānti for three times, we are praying for peace in every level: peace for ourselves, peace for others and peace for the entire creation.

◆ There is only one cause for all mental problems, worries and anxieties: selfishness.

Oṃ śānti：śānti意为和平、太平、平静。Oṃ śānti是两个曼陀罗的结合，为我们提供了一种强烈积极的振动，以及一种全新的能量。当我们唱诵三遍śānti时，我们祈祷每一个层次的和平：我们自身的和平，他人的和平，以及世间万物的和平。

㉑Namaste: Namaste literally means "I bow to you". Usually we place hands together in front of the chest and bow the head while saying namaste.

Namaste: Namaste字面意思为"我向你鞠躬致敬"。通常，我们在说namaste的同时双手合十于胸前并低头致意。

㉒ 对初次见面的服务对象还可以说：

May I help you? （我可以帮您吗？）

Is there anything I can do for you? （有什么我能帮您的吗？）

面对老会员，可以直接进行问候寒暄，比如：

How are you today? （你今天怎么样？）

How is your day? （今天过得如何？）

What's new? （有什么新鲜事吗？）

◆所有精神问题、担忧和焦虑的原因只有一个：自私。

Appendix 2: Simplified Pronunciation of Sanskrit Words
附录2：梵文词汇简化读音

说明：本书对所涉及的瑜伽梵文词汇作了简化转写，并注明变音符号以求发音准确。（参考Swami Satchidananda. *The Yoga Sutras of Patanjali*. Integral Yoga Publications, 2012.）为方便广大读者使用，特引入英文读音供对比学习。对于梵文有严格学习需求的人群，建议在专业梵文老师的指导下学习。

元音部分

（1）单元音

a　类似英语up中的u

ā　同上u音，但保持两倍音长

i　类似英语fill中的i

ī　同上i音，但保持两倍音长

u　类似英语full中的u

ū　同上u音，但保持两倍音长

ṛ　类似英语Christmas中的r

ṝ　同上r音，但保持两倍音长

ḷ　类似英语flip中的l

◆ Accept suffering if it comes. But you need not go looking for pain; you should avoid causing pain either to yourself or to others.

（2）双元音

e　　类似英语they中的e

ai　　类似英语aisle中的ai

o　　类似英语go中的o

au　　类似英语how中的ow

（3）辅助符号

ṃ　　"随韵"（anusvāra），多用于词尾。以m收尾的词，若遇到的下一个词以辅音起首，则m变为鼻化音ṃ。类似英语hum中的m。

ḥ　　"止韵"（visarga），常见于词尾，提示最后一个音为ḥ之前元音的重复，如aḥ听起来是aha，iḥ听起来是ihi。

辅音部分

（1）喉音

k　　类似英语seek中的k

kh　　类似英语back-hand中的k-h

g　　类似英语good中的g

gh　　类似英语dig-hard中的g-h

n　　类似英语sing中的n

（2）腭音

c　　类似英语chum中的ch

◆如果痛苦来了，就接受它。但你不必去寻找痛苦；你应该避免给自己或别人带来痛苦。

ch   类似英语Church-hill中的ch-h

j   类似英语joy中的j

jh   类似英语hedge-hog中的dge-h

ñ   类似英语canyon中的ny

（3）卷舌音

ṭ   类似英语tub中的t

ṭh   类似英语cutting中的tt

ḍ   类似英语deer中的d

ḍh   类似英语red-hot中的d-h

ṇ   类似英语bunting中的n

（4）齿音

t   类似英语pasta中的t

th   类似英语eat honey中的t-h

d   类似英语dense中的d

dh   上述d音向外送气

n   类似英语nut中的n

（5）唇音

p   类似英语pin中的p

ph   类似英语up-hill中的p-h

b   类似英语bird中的b

bh   类似英语abhor中的bh

m   类似英语mud中的m

◆ A person who is totally free from wants will not be like a dummy doing nothing.

瑜伽英语入门指南
附录 | 293

（6）半元音

y　　类似英语yes中的y

r　　类似英语run中的r

l　　类似英语light中的l

v　　类似英语vain中的v

（7）咝音

s　　类似英语sun中的s

ś　　类似英语shut中的sh

ṣ　　类似英语schnapps中的sch

（8）气音

h　　类似英语honey中的h

注：本书中出现了梵文中较为常见的组合音节jña，读音听起来像是ngya（g不发音）。

◆一个完全没有欲望的人不会像无所事事的傻瓜一样。

Appendix 3: List of Yogāsana Names
附录3：瑜伽体式名称索引表

梵文名称	英文译名	中文译名	页码
Adho Mukha Śvānāsana	Downward-facing Dog pose	下犬式	165
Ānanda Bālāsana	Happy Baby pose	快乐婴儿式	139
Ardha Matsyendrāsana	Half Lord-of-the-fish pose	半鱼王式	169
Ardha Padmāsana	Half-lotus pose	半莲花盘坐	255
Āshwa Sañchalanāsana	Equestrian pose	骑马式	193
Aṣṭāṅga Namaskāra	Eight-limbed Salutation pose	八体投地式	113
Baddha Koṇāsana	Bound Angle pose	束角式	99
Bhujaṅgāsana	Cobra pose	眼镜蛇式	197
Bītilāsana	Cow pose	牛式	163
Daṇḍāsana	Staff pose	手杖式	79
Dhanurāsana	Bow pose	弓式	125
Garuḍāsana	Eagle pose	鹰式	73
Gomukhāsana	Cow-face pose	牛面式	95
Halāsana	Plow pose	犁式	147
Hasta Utthānāsana	Raised Arms pose	展臂式	191

◆ Desires for the benefits of others do not create further desires. But personal desires constantly create others, which do not allow the mind to remain calm.

续表

梵文名称	英文译名	中文译名	页码
Jānu Śīrṣāsana	Head-to-knee pose	单腿头碰膝式	83
Makarāsana	Crocodile pose	鳄鱼式	109
Maṇḍūkāsana	Frog pose	青蛙式	129
Mārjāriāsana	Cat Stretch pose	猫伸展式	161
Pādahastāsana	Hand-to-foot pose	手至脚式	193
Padmāsana	Full-lotus pose	全莲花盘坐	255
Paripūrṇa Nāvāsana	Complete Boat pose	完全船式	175
Parvatāsana	The Summit pose	顶峰式	195
Paśchimottānāsana	Seated Forward Bend pose	坐立前屈式	89
Pāvānamuktāsana	Wind-relieving pose	排气式	143
Pranāmāsana	Prayer pose	祈祷式	189
Śalabhāsana	Locust pose	蝗虫式	121
Śavāsana	Corpse pose	挺尸式	155
Setubandhāsana	Bridge pose	桥式	179
Sukhāsana	Easy pose	简易坐	255
Supta Vīrāsana	Reclining Hero pose	仰卧英雄式	151
Sūrya Namaskāra	Sun Salutation	瑜伽拜日式	187
Tāḍāsana	Mountain pose	山式	41

◆为他人谋利的欲望不会产生进一步的欲望。但是个人私欲会不断地产生其他欲望，而这些欲望令头脑无法保持平静。

续表

梵文名称	英文译名	中文译名	页码
Upaviṣṭha Koṇāsana	Seated Angle pose	坐角式	105
Uṣṭrāsana	Camel pose	骆驼式	183
Utkaṭāsana	Chair pose	幻椅式	51
Utthita Trikoṇāsana	Extended Triangle pose	三角伸展式	55
Viparīta Karaṇī	Legs-up-the-wall pose	靠墙倒剪式	135
Vīrabhadrāsana I	Warrior pose I	战士一式	67
Vṛkṣāsana	Tree pose	树式	63

注:

瑜伽体式名称的表述目前在国内仍未达到统一,但这些名称的表述也是有规律可循的。据笔者个人观察,广泛使用的瑜伽体式命名方式大概分为两类。一类是梵文译为英文后,从英文直译为中文。这种体式名称基本保留了原有梵文的意义,属于命名较为准确的一类,如树式——Vṛkṣāsana(vṛkṣa—tree—树;āsana—pose—体式)。另外一类是拟态类,即体式名称描述体式的样态,但含义往往与原来的梵文意义不再相关。比较典型的是幻椅式——Utkaṭāsana。utkaṭa在梵文中意为fierce(凶猛的,猛烈的),而目前广泛使用的名称则模拟其体式形象,将Utkaṭāsana英译为Chair pose(椅子式),中文译名则在这个英文译名的基础上有了进一步发挥,称该体式为"幻椅式"(从中文译到英文写成Imaginary Chair pose,想象或幻想出来的椅子)。

◆ If selfish desires are fulfilled, you swing to the positive side which is called excitement; if unfulfilled, you swing to the negative side, depression. But with selfless desires, you don't swing with the results; you always enjoy what you are doing.

Appendix 4: List of Sanskrit Terms
附录4：梵文词汇表

梵文（注音）	英文释义	中文释义
abhiniveśa	fear of death	畏死
anāhata cakra	heart cakra	心轮
āsana	pose, posture	体式
aṣṭāṅga	eight-limbs	阿斯汤加（八肢）
asmitā	egoism	自我
ātman	the Supreme Soul	至尊灵魂
avidyā	ignorance	无明
āyāma	control, expansion	控制，扩展
bandha	bondage, lock	束缚，锁
bhakti	devotion	奉献
cakra	"wheel", energy centre	"轮"，能量中心，脉轮
dhāraṇā	concentration	专注
dhyāna	meditation	冥想
dveṣa	hatred	憎恶
haṭha	union of the solar and lunar energy	阴阳能量相合，哈达
iḍā	left nāḍī (feminine, lunar)	左脉（阴性的）
Jālandhāra Bandha	throat lock	喉锁
jñāna	knowledge, wisdom	智慧
Jñāna mudrā	gesture of wisdom	智慧手印
karma	action	行动
kleśa	obstacle, affliction	障碍，苦恼
kuṇḍalinī	energy which moves up the body through the suṣumnā nāḍī	体内经由中脉向上的能量，昆达里尼

◆如果自私的欲望得到满足，你会转向积极的一面，即兴奋；如果没有得到满足，你就会转向消极的一面，沮丧。但有了无私的欲望，你就不会随着结果摇摆不定；你会一直享受自己所做的事情。

续表

梵文（注音）	英文释义	中文
Mahā Bandha	the great lock	大收束法
maṇipūra cakra	navel cakra	脐轮
mantra	subtle sound vibration, incantation	精微音振，咒语
Mūla Bandha	perineum contraction	根锁（会阴收束）
mudrā	seal	封印
mūlādhāra cakra	root cakra	根轮
nāḍī	energy channel	能量通道，纳迪
Nāḍī śodhana	purification or cleansing of the nāḍīs	对能量通道的净化或清洁
namaste	I bow to you	我向你鞠躬致敬
nidrā	deep, dreamless sleep	深度、无梦睡眠
niyama	observance	劝制
Om	or written as AUM	初始之音
piṅgalā	right nāḍī (masculine, solar)	右脉（阳性的）
prāṇa	vital energy force	生命之气
prāṇāyāma	regulation of breath	调息
pratyāhāra	sense withdrawal	制感
ragā	attachment	贪恋
rāja	king	王
sahasrāra cakra	crown cakra	顶轮
samādhi	super-conscious state	超意识状态，三摩地
śānti	peace	和平
suṣumnā	central nāḍī (neutral)	中脉（中性的）
svādhiṣṭhāna cakra	sacral cakra	骶骨轮
Uḍḍīyāna Bandha	abdominal contraction	腹锁（腹部收束）
viśuddha cakra	throat cakra	喉轮
yama	abstinence	禁制
yoga	yoke, union	结合，联合，瑜伽

◆ Don't hoard things—having more than you need. You won't know which to use, where to keep them, or how to take care of them.

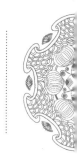

［1］Atré, Zubin. *It Takes Two to Yoga: Asanas for Coups and Partners*. Rupa Publications, 2016.

［2］Ahlund, Jan. *The Yoga Toolbox: An Everyday Guide for Shaping Your Life*. Babaji's Kriya Yoga and Publications, 2010.

［3］Ashley-Farrand, Thomas. *Healing Mantras*: *Using Sound Affirmations for Personal Power, Creativity, and Healing*. Ballantine Wellspring, 1999.

［4］Bachman, Nicolai. *The Language of Yoga: Complete A-Y Guide to Asana Names, Sanskrit Terms, and Chants*. Sounds True Inc, 2005.

［5］Clark, Bernie. *The Complete Guide to Yin Yoga: The Philosophy and Practice of Yin Yoga*. White Cloud Press, 2012.

［6］Clennell, Bobby. *The Women's Yoga Book: Asana and*

◆不要囤积东西——拥有比你所需更多的东西。你会不知道该用哪一个，把它们放在哪里，或者如何打理它们。

Pranayama for all Phases of the Menstrual Cycle. Rodmell Press, 2007.

[7] Desai, Kamini. *Yoga Nidrā: The Art of Transformational Sleep.* Lotus Press, 2017.

[8] Eliot, Travis. *A Journey into Yin Yoga.* Human Kinetics Inc, 2017.

[9] Fishman, Loren. *Healing Yoga: Proven Postures to Treat Twenty Common Ailments—from Backache to Bone Loss, Shoulder Pain to Bunions, and More.* W. W. Norton & Company, 2015.

[10] Joseph and Lilian Le Page. *Yoga Toolbox for Teachers and Students (3rd edition).* Integrative Yoga Therapy, 2015.

[11] Iyengar, B.K.S. *Iyengar Yoga: The Path to Holistic Health.* DK Publishing, 2014.

[12] Iyengar, B.K.S. *Yoga Wisdom and Practice—For Health, Happiness and a Better World.* DK Publishing, 2009.

[13] Iyengar, B.K.S. *Light on Yoga: The Bible of Modern Yoga.* Schocken Books, 1995.

[14] Iyengar, Geeta S. *Yoga in Action: Intermediate Course-I.* YOG, 2013.

[15] Iyengar, Geeta S. *The Tree of Yoga.* Shambhala Publications, 2002.

[16] Iyengar, Geeta S. *Yoga in Action: Preliminary Course.* YOG, 2000.

[17] Iyengar, Geeta S. *Yoga: A Gem for Women.* Timeless Books, 1995.

◆ Selfless people are the most peaceful. They express their state of peace and remain in it by performing every action just for the sake of the action; that is, not expecting one thing in return, not even appreciation.

［18］Kaivalya, Alanna. *Sacred Sound: Discovering the Myth and Meaning of Mantra and Kirtan*. New World Library, 2014.

［19］Langford, Kevin. *Anatomy 101*. Adams Media, 2015.

［20］Mader, Sylvia. *Understanding Human Anatomy & Physiology*. McGraw-Hill, 2005.

［21］Miller, Richard. *Yoga Nidrā: A Meditative Practice for Deep Relaxation and Healing*. Sounds True Inc, 2010.

［22］Stephens, Mark. *Teaching Yoga: Essential Foundations and Techniques*. North Atlantic Books, 2010.

［23］Muktibodhananda, Swami. *Hatha Yoga Pradipika: Light on Hatha Yoga*. Yoga Publications Trust, 2006.

［24］Narayanananda, Swami. *The Secrets of Prana, Pranayama & Yoga-Asanas*. N. K. Prasad & Company, 1959.

［25］Nirmalananda Giri. *Om Yoga: Its Theory and Practice*. Atma Jyoti Press, 2006.

［26］Osho. *A Course in Meditation: A 21-Day Workout for Your Consciousness*. Harmony Books, 2019.

［27］Satchidananda, Swami. *Integral Yoga Hatha for Beginners*. Integral Yoga Publications, 2009.

［28］Satchidananda, Swami. *The Yoga Sutras of Patanjali*. Integral Yoga Publications, 2008.

［29］Satchidananda, Swami. *To Know Your Self*. Integral Yoga Publications, 2008.

［30］Satchidananda, Swami. *Beyond Words*. Integral Yoga Publications, 2008.

◆无私的人是最平静的。他们只是为了行动而行动，以此来表达自己的和平状态并保持在其中；也就是说，不求任何回报，甚至不求感激。

［31］Satchidananda, Swami. *Integral Yoga Hatha for Pregnant Women*. Integral Yoga Publications, 1997.

［32］Satyananda Saraswati, Swami. *Meditation from the Tantras*. Yoga Publications Trust, 2018.

［33］Satyananda Saraswati, Swami. *Asana Pranayama Mudra Bandha*. Yoga Publications Trust, 2013.

［34］Satyananda Saraswati, Swami. *Yoga Nidrā*. Yoga Publications Trust, 2013.

［35］Satyananda Saraswati, Swami. *Surya Namaskara: A Technique of Solar Vitalization*. Yoga Publications Trust, 2011.

［36］Sivananda, Swami. *Amrita Gita*. A Divine Life Society Publication, 1999.

［37］Sivananda, Swami. *Practical Lessons in Yoga*. A Divine Life Society Publication, 1997.

［38］Sivananda, Swami. *The Science of Pranayama*. A Divine Life Society Publication, 1997.

［39］Szcześniak, Konrad & Porzuczek, Andrzej. *Transcription Practice for the International Phonetic Alphabet: Exercises for Students of English*. Cambridge Scholars Publishing, 2020.

［40］Yogakanti, Swami. *Sanskrit Glossary of Yogic Terms*. Yoga Publications Trust, 2007.

［41］*Chinese-English Visual Bilingual Dictionary*. Dorling Kindersley Limited, 2008.

［42］徐娜娜：《体式神话：瑜伽传统故事精粹》，四川人民出版社，2020年。

◆ Choose whatever you like—but do it.

［43］王东旭、吴华军：《瑜伽梵语实用手册》，四川人民出版社，2018年。

［44］《健身瑜伽体位标准（试行）》，国家体育总局社会体育指导中心审定，2018年。

［45］斯瓦米·萨特亚南达·萨拉斯瓦提：《体位法 调息法 契合法 收束法》，东北大学出版社，2015年。

［46］霍恩比：牛津高阶英汉双语词典（第七版），商务印书馆，2009年。

［47］汪文珍：《英语语音》，上海外语教育出版社，2005年。

［48］https://www.yogajournal.com.au.

［49］http://youdao.com/.

［50］http://www.beita.org/html/xianguanzhuangyanlunxuexi/fanwenxuexi/200901/25-1718.html.

◆选择任何你喜欢的——但要去做。

图书在版编目（ＣＩＰ）数据

瑜伽英语入门指南 / 徐娜娜著. — 成都：四川人
民出版社，2024.4
ISBN 978-7-220-12882-0

Ⅰ.①瑜…　Ⅱ.①徐…　Ⅲ.①瑜伽—英语—自学参考
资料　Ⅳ.①R161.1

中国国家版本馆CIP数据核字(2023)第014024号

YUJA YINGYU RUMENZHINAN
瑜伽英语入门指南

徐娜娜　著

责任编辑	蒋科兰　孙　茜
封面设计	李秋烨
版式设计	戴雨虹
特约校对	张新伟
责任印制	周　奇
出版发行	四川人民出版社（成都三色路238号）
网　　址	http://www.scpph.com
E-mail	scrmcbs@sina.com
新浪微博	@四川人民出版社
微信公众号	四川人民出版社
发行部业务电话	（028）86361653　86361656
防盗版举报电话	（028）86361653
照　　排	成都木之雨文化传播有限公司
印　　刷	四川五洲彩印有限责任公司
成品尺寸	146mm×208mm
印　　张	10.5
字　　数	210 千字
版　　次	2024 年 4 月第 1 版
印　　次	2024 年 4 月第 1 次印刷
书　　号	ISBN 978-7-220-12882-0
定　　价	52.00元